Student Study Guide to Accompany

PSYCHIATRIC MENTAL HEALTH NURSING

2nd EDITION

Student Study Guide to Accompany
PSYCHIATRIC MENTAL HEALTH NURSING

2nd EDITION

Noreen Cavan Frisch, RN, PhD, FAAN
Professor and Chair
Department of Nursing
Cleveland State University
Cleveland, Ohio

Lawrence E. Frisch, MPH, PhD
Department of Preventive Medicine
The University of Kansas School of Medicine—Wichita
Wichita, Kansas

Prepared by
Ruth A. Griffin, RN, MSN
Doctoral Student in Nursing
Columbia University
New York, New York

DELMAR

THOMSON LEARNING

Australia Canada Mexico Singapore Spain United Kingdom United States

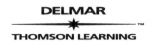

DELMAR

THOMSON LEARNING

Student Study Guide to Accompany
Psychiatric Mental Health Nursing, 2nd Edition
Noreen Cavan Frisch and Lawrence E. Frisch

Business Unit Director:
William Brottmiller

Executive Editor:
Cathy L. Esperti

Acquisitions Editor:
Mathew Kane

Developmental Editor:
Marjorie A. Bruce

Editorial Assistant:
Shelley Esposito

Executive Marketing Manager:
Dawn F. Gerrain

Channel Manager:
Tara Carter

Project Editor:
Maureen M. E. Grealish

Production Coordinator:
Nina Lontrato

Art/Design Coordinator:
Robert Plante

NOTICE TO THE READER

Contents

UNIT 3: SPECIAL POPULATIONS

UNIT 4: NURSING INTERVENTIONS AND TREATMENT MODALITIES

UNIT 5: CARING FOR THE NURSE

Preface

The purpose of the *Student Study Guide to Accompany Psychiatric Mental Health Nursing* is to help you learn, absorb, and retain difficult and often unfamiliar concepts in psychiatric nursing. Although this *Study Guide* will not serve as a substitute for reading *Psychiatric Mental Health Nursing*, it will help reinforce the major concepts as you review the central facts of each chapter and suggest study strategies that will help you retain the material, perform well on tests, and develop the psychiatric knowledge and skills you will need to succeed as a nurse in any health care setting.

Each chapter of the *Study Guide* covers three areas: key terms, exercises and activities, and self-assessment.

Key Terms

The language of psychiatric nursing is specialized and sometimes difficult. Avoid the temptation to skip over this element in the textbook and in the *Study Guide*. Learning how to use this potent and interesting language will enhance your performance in the course and increase your effectiveness as a nurse. As a nurse, you need to be able to explain these concepts to your clients and their families, and you need to use these terms correctly and easily in your communication with your colleagues and other health professionals. The best time to learn terminology is the first time you encounter it.

Exercises and Activities

The Exercises and Activities sections identify the key concepts in the textbook chapters and challenge you to relate the concepts of psychiatric nursing to your own life and experience. There is no better teacher than your own experience. If you can relate the textbook content to your own life, to people you have known, even to movies and television shows you have seen, and to books you have read, the knowledge will be personal and meaningful to you.

Self-Assessment Quizzes

If you can answer the test questions in the self-test correctly and confidently, then you have mastered most of the essential content of these chapters. The Self-Assessment Quizzes offer a great way to test your knowledge strengths and weaknesses.

The combination of *Psychiatric Mental Health Nursing* and this *Study Guide*, along with your clinical exposure, your instructor, and your classmates, should make this course in psychiatric nursing an intensely personal and rewarding experience for you. Psychiatric nursing may or may not have been what attracted you to nursing in the first place. However, it is our hope that what you gain from this experience will enhance your effectiveness as a nurse in ways you could never have imagined before this term began.

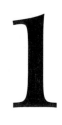

Through the Door: Your First Day in Psychiatric Nursing

The purpose of this chapter is to explore your own feelings and attitudes toward psychiatric mental health nursing. The chapter offers strategies for coping in the strange new world of psychiatric nursing. It helps you anticipate some of the role changes and rites of passage ahead of you in this course.

Reading Assignment

Please read Chapter 1, "Through the Door: Your First Day in Psychiatric Nursing," pages 3–13.

Key Terms

Write definitions for the following terms in your own words. Compare your definitions with those given in the text on page 4.

Depression _____

_____

Disability _____

_____

Distress _____

_____

Hallucination _____

_____

Mania _____

_____

Mental Disorder _____

_____

Mental Health _____

_____

Mental Illness _____

_____

Psychosis _____

_____

Exercises and Activities

1. Read the chapter opening box on page 3. Answer the following questions in your own words.

   a. What has been your experience with and exposure to psychiatric nursing?

   _____

   _____

   _____

   _____

   _____

   b. What are your ideas and images of psychiatry and mental health care? Where do they come from?

   _____

   _____

   _____

   _____

   _____

   c. What are your feelings about taking a course in psychiatric mental health nursing? Are you anxious? Interested? Curious?

   _____

   _____

   _____

   _____

   _____

2. Brainstorm a list of your own personality traits and personal characteristics. Arrange them in two columns labeled *Mentally Healthy* and *Mentally Unhealthy*.

Mentally Healthy	Mentally Unhealthy
_____	_____
_____	_____
_____	_____
_____	_____

Take a critical look at the results. Are you satisfied with the balance?

_____

_____

_____

_____

_____

3. Read "The Parallel Universe," by Susanna Kaysen, on page 7.

   a. Is "parallel universe" a good analogy for mental illness? Why or why not?

   _____

   _____

   _____

   _____

   _____

   b. What does the author mean by: "Every window on Alcatraz has a view of San Francisco"?

   _____

   _____

   _____

   _____

   _____

4. Read the Nursing Tip on page 10.

   a. What should your main focus be when starting a conversation with a psychotic client?

   _____

   _____

   _____

   _____

   _____

b. List some ways you can build rapport with a psychotic client; include both verbal and nonverbal strategies.

_____

_____

_____

_____

_____

c. The authors emphasize the importance of "listening, watching, and being there." What do they mean by "being there"? How might a depressed client respond to your "being there"? Can you think of other nonpsychiatric nursing experiences you've had when "being there" was therapeutic?

_____

_____

_____

_____

_____

5. Read "Student Nurses" on page 10.

a. Does the client's perception and opinion of student nurses surprise you?

_____

_____

_____

_____

b. How do her responses compare to the responses of other clients you have met in nonpsychiatric settings?

_____

_____

_____

_____

6. Start a journal and keep it throughout the course. You might consider writing about certain themes that you can follow through this once-in-a-lifetime learning experience; for example, how your attitude toward mentally ill individuals evolves over time. Also, are there concepts and behaviors you just don't understand? How is your role changing? Will you become more confident of your skills? Who are some of the memorable clients and staff members you have met? What insights will you gain that will make you a better nurse, even in a regular medical setting?

7. Read the "Advice from Prior Students" on page 11. Log on to the Frisch Online Companion (www.DelmarNursing.com) and based on your experience, offer your advice to future students of psychiatric mental health nursing.

8. Try repeating the following affirmations to yourself:

   "I can tolerate a certain amount of ambiguity."

   "Don't be afraid to make a mistake."

   "Mistakes are opportunities to learn."

   "I can trust the staff to look out for me."

   "People respond most positively to me when I am just myself."

   Write some affirmations that are tailored to meet your specific needs as you begin your study of psychiatric mental health nursing.

   _____

   _____

   _____

   _____

   _____

Self-Assessment Quiz

1. Mental health and mental illness are, to some extent, a matter of degrees. (page 6)

   ❑ True

   ❑ False

2. A person can have symptoms of mental illness without being mentally ill. (page 7)

   ❑ True

   ❑ False

3. *Psychosis* means that an individual (page 8)

   a.   suffers from mental retardation.

   b.   has lost the ability to recognize reality.

   c.   experiences bouts of alcoholism.

   d.   is visually impaired.

4. People who are profoundly depressed (page 8)

   a.   display boundless energy.

   b.   talk in a boring monotone.

   c.   may need to be protected against suicidal impulses.

   d.   need rest and relaxation.

5. *Mania* is manifested by the following traits (page 8):

   a.   Remarkable memory

   b.   Smiles and gestures

   c.   Poutiness

   d.   Exaggerated sense of well-being

6. Why do clients with the symptoms of mental illness seek care and treatment? (page 9)

   a.   Self-referral due to experience of pain

   b.   Family, friends, health professionals, and spiritual advisors urge treatment

   c.   Police transport clients to mental health treatment centers

   d.   All of the above

7. Which of the following is not a good strategy when conversing with psychotic clients? (page 10)

   a.   Introduce yourself; then, be yourself.

   b.   Concentrate on the immediate time, place, and situation.

   c.   Use humor to establish rapport.

   d.   Focus on concrete words and topics, rather than abstractions.

8. Although some students wish they didn't have to take psychiatric mental health nursing, the authors suggest benefits every nursing student might derive from this course. These benefits include (pages 5, 10–11):

    a. Discovering you might want to become a psychiatric nurse

    b. Mastering interpersonal skills essential in any nursing setting

    c. Gaining new insights into yourself that will make you a better nurse

    d. All of the above

9. Define "rites of passage." (page 12)

    _____

    _____

    _____

    _____

    _____

10. What do you think the authors mean by the phrase "being present"? (page 11)

    _____

    _____

    _____

    _____

    _____

Psychiatric Nursing: The Evolution of a Specialty

2

The purpose of Chapter 2 is to build a context for how psychiatric nursing developed and why it is needed. Along the way, the chapter identifies some of the pioneers of psychiatric nursing and the major legislation that has led to the modern treatment of mental illnesses.

Reading Assignment

Please read Chapter 2, "Psychiatric Nursing: The Evolution of a Specialty," pages 15–25.

Key Terms

Write definitions for the following terms in your own words. Compare your definitions with those given in the text on page 16.

Asylum_____

_____

Brown Report _____

_____

National Mental Health Act _____

_____

Psychiatric Mental Health Advanced Practice Registered Nurse _____

_____

Psychiatric Mental Health Nurse _____

_____

Exercises and Activities

1. Read the chapter opening box on page 15. Compare and contrast psychiatric nursing to other nursing specialties.

   _____

   _____

   _____

   _____

   _____

2. Read the Reflective Thinking box on page 17.

    a. Who do you think the "deviants" are in our current society?

        _____

        _____

        _____

        _____

        _____

    b. What does the contemporary treatment of mentally ill people say about our society and our values?

        _____

        _____

        _____

        _____

        _____

3. Study Van Gogh's painting on page 19.

    a. What characteristics of the care of the mentally ill in the nineteenth century are depicted in this painting?

        _____

        _____

        _____

        _____

        _____

    b. What observations can you make about the communication taking place in this painting? In what ways would communication be different in a mental health setting today?

        _____

        _____

        _____

        _____

        _____

4. The following events are referenced in Table 2–2 on page 22. To develop a sense of how psychiatric nursing has evolved over the past two centuries, match the year with the important event that took place that year:

_____The National League for Nursing made psychiatric nursing a requirement for accreditation of basic nursing programs

_____Publication of the first psychiatric nursing textbook, *Nursing Mental Diseases*, by Harriet Bailey

_____Publication of *Interpersonal Relations in Nursing* by nurse theorist Hildegard Peplau

_____First mental hospital in the United States established in Williamsburg, Virginia

_____Publication of the Brown Report, which recommended that psychiatric nursing be included in general nursing education

_____First use of the term *psychiatry* by physicians attempting to upgrade the status of their work with the mentally ill

_____Johns Hopkins Hospital included psychiatric nursing in the course of study for general nurses

_____First school for psychiatric nurses (or mental nurses) established at the McLean Asylum in Somerville, Massachusetts

_____Passage of the National Mental Health Act, which established the National Institutes of Mental Health (NIMH)

	1773
	1846
	1882
	1913
	1920
	1946
	1948
	1952
	1955

Check your answers in the text.

5. Create a timeline of important events in the history and practice of psychiatric mental health nursing. Update it throughout the course.

6. Review Table 2-1 on page 18, summarizing theories of mental illness formulated in the nineteenth century. Based on what you know today, what would you call our current understanding of mental illness, and what are its premises? Do you expect your view to evolve during this course?

_____

_____

_____

_____

_____

7. Briefly summarize the contributions of these pioneers of psychiatric nursing:

   a. Dorothea Lynde Dix

   _____

   _____

   _____

   _____

   _____

   b. Isabel Hampton Robb

   _____

   _____

   _____

   _____

   _____

   c. Lavinia Lloyd Dock

   _____

   _____

   _____

   _____

   _____

8. List as many career opportunities for the psychiatric nurse, outside of a locked psychiatric hospital, as you can.

_____

_____

_____

_____

_____

9. Characterize the challenge of the future of psychiatric nursing.

_____

_____

_____

_____

_____

Self-Assessment Quiz

1. Society has almost always viewed mental illnesses as diseases. (page 17)

   ❑ True

   ❑ False

2. Clients of asylums were first called inmates. (page 18)

   ❑ True

   ❑ False

3. Walt Whitman, the American poet who served as a nurse during the Civil War, wrote "Leaves of Grass" to expose the deplorable conditions of the psychiatric institutions of his day. (page 8)

   ❑ True

   ❑ False

4. The National League for Nursing recommended in 1937 that schools of nursing incorporate psychiatric nursing into their curriculum, but didn't require it for accreditation until 1955. (page 21)

   ❑ True

   ❑ False

5. Wars, including the Civil War, World War I, and World War II, produced no increase in the need for mental health services. (pages 18 and 21)

   ❑ True

   ❑ False

6. Of the following, which is not an important publication in the history of psychiatric nursing? (page 21)

   a. "Utilitarianism" by John Stuart Mill

   b. *Nursing Mental Diseases* by Harriet Bailey

   c. *Interpersonal Relations in Nursing* by Hildegard Peplau

   d. The Brown Report by Esther Lucille Brown

7. Nursing training schools were established at leading psychiatric hospitals because (page 21)

   a. the asylums wanted free labor.

   b. there was a need to recruit women to care for people with mental illnesses.

   c. there weren't enough doctors to take care of all the clients.

   d. the Civil War had produced an abundance of mentally ill people.

8. Match the time period in the left-hand column to the prevalence of the treatment modalities in the right-hand column. (pages 17–21)

   _____Ancient times   a. Isolation from society

   _____Middle Ages   b. Reverence or repulsion

   _____Late 1800s   c. Insulin and electric shock

   _____Early 1900s   d. Physical labor

   _____1920s   e. Hot and cold packs

   _____1930s   f. Psychopharmacology

   _____1950s   g. Humane custodial care

9. Match the psychiatric pioneer with his or her unique contribution. (pages 17–21)

_____Hildegard Peplau   a. Early believer in treating mental illness as disease

_____Dorothea Dix   b. Early advocate of training for nurses

_____William Battie   c. First required psychiatric nursing in nursing curriculm

_____Edward Cowles   d. Started formal training for mental nurses

_____Isabel Hampton Robb   e. Advocated affiliation between nursing schools and psychiatric hospitals

_____Effie Taylor

_____Esther Brown   f. Defined nurse-client relationships

g. Advocated humane treatment of the mentally ill

Theory as Basis for Practice

3

The purpose of Chapter 3 is to establish the theoretical basis of psychiatric nursing. After first discussing theories specific to nursing, the chapter discusses the major theories of psychology.

Reading Assignment

Please read Chapter 3, "Theory as Basis for Practice," pages 27–59.

Key Terms

Write definitions for the following terms in your own words. Compare your definitions with those on page 29 in the text.

Adaptive Potential _____

_____

Cognition _____

_____

Concept _____

_____

Conceptual Framework _____

_____

Created Environment _____

_____

Cultural Care _____

_____

Cultural Care Accommodation/Negotiation _____

_____

Cultural Care Preservation/Maintenance _____

_____

Cultural Care Repatterning/Restructuring _____

_____

Culture _____

_____

Ego _____

_____

External Environment _____

_____

Extrapersonal Stressor _____

_____

Fixation _____

_____

Folk System _____

_____

Id _____

_____

Internal Environment _____

_____

Interpersonal Stressor _____

_____

Intrapersonal Stressor _____

_____

Modeling _____

_____

Nursing Agency _____

_____

Nursing Situation _____

_____

Professional System _____

_____

Regression _____

_____

Role-Modeling _____

_____

Self-Care _____

_____

Self-Care Agency _____

_____

Self-Care Deficit _____

_____

Superego _____

_____

Theory _____

_____

Therapeutic Self-Care Demand _____

_____

Exercises and Activities

1. Read the chapter-opening for Chapter 3 on page 27.

    a. Write a definition for the word "theory."

    _____

    _____

    b. How is the word "theory" used in everyday conversation?

    _____

    _____

    _____

    _____

    _____

    c. How is the word "theory" used in a discipline?

    _____

    _____

    _____

    _____

    _____

2. Review the Reflective Thinking box concerning theory on page 31.

    a. Why is theory important to nursing practice?

    _____

    _____

    _____

    _____

    _____

    b. Give examples of how your nursing practice might vary if you moved from one nursing theory to another. Think about a specific client care situation and ask yourself how your response might differ from theory to theory.

    _____

    _____

    _____

    _____

    _____

3. Explain the differences between a Theory, a Concept, and a Conceptual Framework. Which is the most general idea? Give an example of each.

    _____

    _____

    _____

    _____

    _____

4. Name the three stages of the nurse's relationship with the client in Peplau's Interpersonal Relations in Nursing Theory, on page 32. Do you agree that this is a regular pattern in your relationship to your clients? Can you think of examples from your own experience that followed this pattern?

    _____

    _____

    _____

    _____

    _____

5. The authors identify four general classes of nursing theories:

   1. Theories based on relationships

   2. Theories based on caring

   3. Theories based on energy fields

   4. Theories based on "when nursing is needed"

      a. Match the classes of theories with the theorists below by identifying which class of theories applies to each theorist

         _____Leininger

         _____Parse

         _____Betty Neuman

         _____Roy

         _____Rogers

         _____Orem

         _____Margaret Newman

         _____Watson

         _____Peplau

         _____Boykin and Shoenhofer

         _____Erickson, Tomlin, and Swain

6. Identify the psychological theorists based on their identification of the ages and stages of man:

   a. _____Trust vs. Mistrust; Autonomy vs. Shame and Doubt; Initiative vs. Guilt; Industry vs. Inferiority; Identity vs. Role Confusion; Intimacy vs. Isolation; Generativity vs. Stagnation; Ego Integrity vs. Despair

   b. _____Sensorimotor Intelligence; Preoperational Thought; Concrete Operations; Formal Operations

   c. _____Physiological Needs; Safety and Security; Love and Belonging; Esteem and Self-esteem; Self-actualization

   d. _____Oral Stage; Anal Stage; Phallic Stage; Latency Age; Puberty

7. Explain how nursing theories and psychological theories can work together. Do nursing theories account for human development and explain mental illness? Do psychological theories offer guidance on nursing practice?

    _____

    _____

    _____

    _____

    _____

8. What similarities do you see between Watson's nursing theory and Maslow's developmental theory?

    _____

    _____

    _____

    _____

    _____

9. What similarities do you see between Orem's nursing theory and existential philosophy?

    _____

    _____

    _____

    _____

    _____

10. Review the Reflective Thinking box about sociocultural perspective on page 55.

    a. List the nursing theories you think reflect a more sociocultural perspective.

        _____

        _____

        _____

        _____

        _____

b. List those that tend to view the individual in isolation of his sociocultural surroundings.

_____

_____

_____

_____

_____

c. Divide the psychological development theories in like manner.

_____

_____

_____

_____

_____

d. Do you see any similarities between the nursing theories and psychological theories that place people in a sociocultural context?

_____

_____

_____

_____

_____

e. Do you see any similarities between the nursing theory and psychological theories that attempt to understand individuals apart from their contextual surroundings?

_____

_____

_____

_____

_____

11. Read the Reflective Thinking box on page 56 about the "myth" of mental illness. Considering that definitions and responses to mental illness throughout history have changed and evolved, is it possible that our current conception of mental illness is wrong? Is the current view of mental illness just a reflection of the twentieth century's obsession with science, rationality, and medical advances? How would you refute Szasz's arguments?

_____

_____

_____

_____

_____

Self-Assessment Quiz

1. No matter what theory is used to guide the nurse's practice in interacting with Mr. James in the chapter's case study (page 31), the recommendation is that Mr. James find new useful ways to use his skills and meet his need for feeling useful and connected to others.

   ❏ True

   ❏ False

2. Theories and conceptual frameworks are pretty much interchangeable terms. (page 30)

   ❏ True

   ❏ False

3. Concepts are the building blocks of theories. (page 30)

   ❏ True

   ❏ False

4. Existentialism emphasizes choice as opposed to the predetermined nature of some earlier psychological theories.

   ❏ True

   ❏ False

5. The superego is the same thing as the conscience. (page 45)

   ❏ True

   ❏ False

6. Neither Freud nor Piaget explain the ages and stages of adulthood. (page 50)

   ❑ True

   ❑ False

7. Skinner tried to show that humans behave in much the same way as pigeons and rats. (pages 54–55)

   ❑ True

   ❑ False

8. Hildegard Peplau's nursing theory is based on therapeutic _____. (page 32)

9. The key concept associated with Erickson, Tomlin, and Swain's nursing theory is _____. (page 32)

10. Two nursing theories based on caring were developed by _____ and _____. (page 34)

11. Rogers, Parse, and Newman developed nursing theories based on _____ _____. (page 38)

12. Orem's theory is known as _____ _____ _____. (page 41)

13. Freud identified three aspects of the personality, which he termed _____, _____, and _____. (page 45)

14. The psychological theorist most closely associated with the ages and stages of man is _____. (pages 51–52)

15. Harry Stack Sullivan believed that people grow psychologically in the context of their _____ relationships. (pages 47–48)

16. Piaget is associated with the _____ development of children. (pages 48–49)

17. Skinner is classified as a _____ psychologist. (page 54)

18. To a nurse who bases her practice on theory, which of the following is not an advantage? (page 31)

    a. being able to more easily transfer knowledge and experience from one situation to another

    b. being able to communicate about nursing practice to others

    c. being able to judge appropriateness of behavior in specific circumstances

    d. being able to practice on the same plane as physicians and pharmacists

19. Sociocultural Theory holds that (page 55)

    a. there is no such thing as mental illness.

    b. society may be "sicker" than its individuals.

    c. culture, society, government, laws, regions, and the economy can all contribute to mental illness.

    d. government programs can be designed to prevent or lessen the severity of mental illness.

Neuroscience as a Basis for Practice

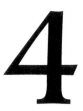

The purpose of Chapter 4 is to establish the theoretical basis of psychiatric nursing. This chapter discusses the contemporary view of the biological basis of mental illness. It may seem odd at first to think of consciousness, emotions, and thoughts in terms of biological processes going on in the nervous and regulatory systems. However, in this chapter, we explore the methodology and findings associated with the relationship between neuroscience and behavior.

Reading Assignment

Please read Chapter 4, "Neuroscience as a Basis for Practice," pages 61–77.

Key Terms

Write definitions for the following terms in your own words. Compare your definitions with those given in the text on page 62.

Computerized Tomography _____

_____

Cortex _____

_____

Diencephalon _____

_____

DNA _____

_____

Genetic Marker _____

_____

Genome _____

_____

Hypothalamus _____

_____

Magnetic Resonance Imaging _____

_____

Neurotransmitter _____

_____

Positron Emission Tomography _____

_____

Synapse _____

_____

Thalamus _____

_____

Exercises and Activities

1. Refer to the discussion of brain anatomy in Figure 4-1 on page 64.

    a. What are the four main divisions of the central nervous system?

    _____

    _____

    _____

    _____

    b. Which of these is related to consciousness and psychiatric disorders?

    _____

    c. Identify the importance, in terms of behavior, of the thalamus and the hypothalamus.

    _____

    _____

    _____

    _____

    _____

    d. Identify the four lobes of the cortex and explain their functions and significance.

    _____

    _____

    _____

    _____

    _____

2. Define "biopsychophysiological theory." (page 63)

_____

_____

_____

_____

_____

   a. How is this theory different from the "classic" theories of psychology and their explanations of mental illness?

       _____

       _____

       _____

       _____

       _____

   b. What similarities and differences do you see between Skinner's behavioral theory and the biopsychophysiological theory?

       _____

       _____

       _____

       _____

       _____

3. The hypothalamus controls the autonomic nervous system. Explain how it regulates changes in our bodies when we experience anxiety.

_____

_____

_____

_____

_____

4. Identify the three major brain imaging technologies and briefly describe the unique
    advantages of each. (pages 66–68)

    _____

    _____

    _____

    _____

    _____

5. Study the material on electrophysiology and neurochemistry on pages 68–72.

    a. Label the structures of the microanatomy of a neuron, reproduced below.

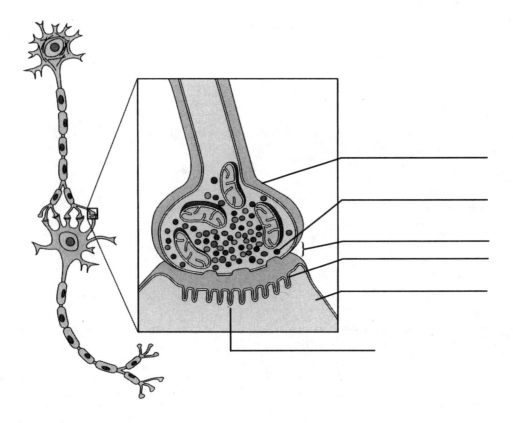

b. State the sequence of events that nerve cells undergo in the process of passing information from one cell to the next.

_____

_____

_____

_____

_____

c. Did the discussion of electrophysiology give you any additional insights into the "energy field" nursing theories discussed in the beginning of this chapter? What are they?

_____

_____

_____

_____

_____

6. Study the section on neurotransmitters on page 72.

a. What characterizes substances as neurotransmitters?

_____

_____

_____

_____

_____

b. Describe the basic mechanism of all neurotransmitters.

_____

_____

_____

_____

_____

c. What is the difference between excitatory stimulation and inhibitory stimulation?

_____

_____

_____

_____

_____

d. How do neurons "know" whether to fire their own action potentials in the presence of numerous neurotransmitters?

_____

_____

_____

_____

_____

7. What recent discovery about membrane receptors explains why clozapine, unlike typical neuroleptic drugs, blocks delusions and hallucinations without causing side effects that resemble Parkinson's disease?

_____

_____

_____

_____

_____

8. What is the relationship between DNA, RNA, and proteins that comprise amino acids?

_____

_____

_____

_____

_____

9. What is the significance of mapping the human genome for the understanding and treatment of mental illness?

_____

_____

_____

_____

_____

Self-Assessment Quiz

1. Biopsychophysiology involves the study of all of the following except

    a. biochemistry.

    b. genetics.

    c. neuroanatomy.

    d. anthropology.

2. The diencephalon includes

    a. the thyroid and the thalamus.

    b. the thyroid and the parathyroid.

    c. the thalamus and the hypothalamus.

    d. the hypothalamus and the pituitary.

3. Structures in the brain connected with the production of memories and emotions include

    a. the limbic system, the amygdala, the hypothalamus, and the cortex.

    b. the limbic system, the amygdala, the hypothalamus, and the optic nerve.

    c. the limbic system, the auditory nerve, the hypothalamus, and the cortex.

    d. the amygdala, the hypothalamus, the cortex, and the optic nerve.

4. Which of the following is not an imaging technology? (pages 66–68)

    a. Computerized tomography

    b. Magnetic resonance imaging

    c. Primal scream therapy

    d. Positron emission tomography

5. Name the four lobes of the cortex. (page 65)

    a. Prefrontal, frontal, parietal, and occipital

    b. Frontal, temporal, spatial, and parietal

    c. Frontal, temporal, occipital, and parietal

    d. Frontal, temporal, occular, and precipital

6. All of the following statements about synapses are true except:

    a. Synapses are very wide compared to gap junctions.

    b. The mechanisms of transmission across synapses is much less complex than those governing transmission across gap junctions.

    c. Ions don't flow across synapses.

    d. Most psychiatric medications act upon the nerve synapses.

7. All of the following statements about neurotransmitters are true except:

    a. Neurotransmitters either excite or inhibit a dentrite.

    b. Neurotransmitters don't cross synaptic clefts.

    c. Neurotransmitters can be controlled precisely by reuptake into the axon that released them.

    d. Many psychiatric drugs prevent the reuptake of neurotransmitters.

8. Tracts differ from nerves in that tracts do not leave the nervous system.

    ❑ True

    ❑ False

9. The human genome is a gene that has been associated with a genetic disease.

    ❑ True

    ❑ False

10. Mutations result when an error takes place in the way a piece of DNA is translated.

    ❑ True

    ❑ False

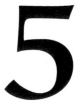

Diagnostic Systems for Psychiatric Nursing

The purpose of this chapter is to explain the various systems for labeling and classifying mental disorders, both from a medical and a nursing standpoint, showing how medical and nursing systems interact. The purposes of these systems are explained, and issues like privacy, confidentiality, and communications among health professionals are explored.

Reading Assignment

Please read Chapter 5, "Diagnostic Systems for Psychiatric Nursing," pages 79–95.

Key Terms

Write definitions for the following terms in your own words. Compare your definitions with those given in the text on page 80.

Classification _____

_____

DSM-IV-TR _____

_____

ICD _____

_____

NANDA _____

_____

NIC _____

_____

NMDS _____

_____

SNOMED_____

_____

UMLS _____

_____

Exercises and Activities

1. Prior to reading this chapter, how familiar were you with the language and systems of psychiatric nursing? Have you used some of these terms before? Were you using the language correctly? Write down areas in which the chapter clarified, corrected, or sharpened your previous knowledge of this specialized language.

   _____

   _____

   _____

   _____

   _____

2. Describe the purpose of each of the following diagnostic systems:

   a. DSM _____

   _____

   b. ICD _____

   _____

   c. NANDA _____

   _____

3. Read the case study of "Maria" on page 82.

   a. Would you know which classification system to use when caring for Maria?

   _____

   b. Would you use more than one classification system? Which ones, and why?

   _____

   _____

   _____

   _____

   _____

4. Review the DSM Axial Diagnoses box for the case example, "Maria," on page 83.

   a. Do you agree with the diagnoses, based on the information given?

   _____

b. Explain why "recent divorce" would be included under Axis IV.

_____

_____

_____

_____

_____

5. Review Table 5-1, "Global Assessment of Functioning Scale," on page 84.

a. Do you agree with the score of 60 assigned to Maria in the case example? Why or why not?

_____

_____

_____

_____

_____

b. Rate another client you have recently encountered, using the GAF Scale. Explain the rationale for your assessment.

_____

_____

_____

_____

_____

c. Would you find this scale useful in your nursing experience? List the advantages and the drawbacks as you see them.

_____

_____

_____

_____

_____

6. Review the Nursing Alert on "Cultural Sensitivity and DSM" on page 85.

    a. Explain why cultural issues might be important to consider before arriving at a psychiatric diagnosis.

    _____

    _____

    _____

    _____

    _____

    b. Do you believe that, ultimately, diagnostic criteria transcend cultural differences? Why or why not?

    _____

    _____

    _____

    _____

    _____

7. Explain why the American Psychiatric Association updated the DSM to "DSM-IV-TR in 2000. How would you characterize the changes?

    _____

    _____

    _____

    _____

    _____

8. Review the Reflective Thinking box on the "Pros and Cons of a Psychiatric Diagnostic System," on page 85.

    a. Do you think a psychiatric center could function effectively without diagnostic systems? How would it function differently if there were no psychiatric diagnostic systems?

    _____

    _____

    _____

    _____

    _____

b. Respond to the following statement: "A nurse should be able to respond therapeutically to a client's behavior without having to categorize or label a client with a diagnosis."

_____

_____

_____

_____

_____

9. Review the Reflective Thinking box, "What Is Unnamed Is Unnoticed," on page 86.

a. How would you respond to a client who displays:

Self-esteem disturbance

_____

_____

_____

_____

_____

Powerlessness

_____

_____

_____

_____

_____

Sleep-pattern disturbance

_____

_____

_____

_____

_____

b.   What strategies would you use to interact with this client?

_____

_____

_____

_____

_____

c.   Provide a sample documentation of the client's diagnosis and your interventions.

_____

_____

_____

_____

_____

10.   Review the "Stages of NANDA Diagnoses" in the box on page 87.

a.   Summarize the changes in the four stages.

_____

_____

_____

_____

_____

b.   What, if any, implications might the stage of a diagnosis have on your clinical utilization of it?

_____

_____

_____

_____

_____

11. Read the Reflective Thinking box, "Are Nursing Diagnoses Useful?", on page 90.

    a. In your own words, state your attitude toward nursing diagnoses.

    _____

    _____

    _____

    _____

    _____

    b. How are you expected to use nursing diagnoses in this course?

    _____

    _____

    _____

    _____

    _____

    c. State the rationale for the way nursing diagnoses are used in this course, and comment on their professional value.

    _____

    _____

    _____

    _____

    _____

12. Review Table 5-2, "Diagnoses from Three Systems for Case Example: Maria," on page 91.

    a. Which of these diagnoses is most useful to you in planning your nursing care?

    _____

    _____

    _____

    _____

    _____

b. Do any of these diagnoses give you so little information that you can't use them in planning nursing care?

_____

13. Review the discussion of the Health Insurance Portability and Accountability Act of 1996, on page 93.

a. What are the provisions and requirement of the Act?

_____

_____

_____

_____

_____

b. What are the drawbacks and loopholes of the Act?

_____

_____

_____

_____

_____

c. How do you expect HIPPA to affect the nursing profession?

_____

_____

_____

_____

_____

14. Read the material on pages 93–94 related to recent advances in diagnostic nomenclature.

a. Write out the full meanings of these acronyms:

UMLS _____

_____

SNOMED _____

_____

NMDS _____

_____

    b. What implications would these advances have for your daily nursing practice?

_____

_____

_____

_____

_____

15. Obtain a copy of the journal *Nursing Diagnosis* and review the articles and issues discussed. What relevance do the issues in this journal have to the way you want to practice nursing?

_____

_____

_____

_____

_____

16. Explain how the Nursing Outcomes Classification (NOC) is structured.

_____

_____

_____

_____

_____

Self-Assessment Quiz

1. ICD-9 is a classification system that defines mental disorders and is multiaxial. (pages 81–82)

   ❏ True

   ❏ False

2. Classification is a system of categorization that allows useful distinctions to be established that may lead to deeper understanding of natural phenomena. (page 81)

   ❏ True

   ❏ False

3. In the DSM-III, Axis I identifies clinical disorders, and Axis II identifies personality disorders and conditions of mental retardation. This is a complete description of the DSM-III Classification System. (page 83)

   ❏ True

   ❏ False

4. The DSM-IV serves as the current "gold standard" for making a mental health diagnosis. (page 85)

   ❏ True

   ❏ False

5. In the GAF Scale, the higher a client scores in the 0–100 range, the lower the client's functioning. (page 83)

   ❏ True

   ❏ False

6. The NANDA nursing diagnoses are used only in psychiatric mental health nursing. (page 86)

   ❏ True

   ❏ False

7. A NANDA diagnosis consists of its name, its definition, a statement of its etiology, and its defining characteristics. (page 87)

   ❏ True

   ❏ False

8. NIC stands for Nursing Interventions Classification. (page 91)

   ❑ True

   ❑ False

9. NIC is used to identify clinical tasks, or activities, that can be carried out by non-nurse multiskilled health workers to assist in the client's treatment program. (page 91)

   ❑ True

   ❑ False

10. All the following are widely used client diagnostic systems: ICD, NANDA, NIC, DSM, NDMS. (page 81)

    ❑ True

    ❑ False

11. As we move closer to a uniform diagnostic system and computerized health records, some of the issues nurses should be concerned about include privacy, confidentiality, and loss of individuality.

    ❑ True

    ❑ False

Tools of Psychiatric Mental Health Nursing: Communication, Nursing Process, and the Nurse-Client Relationship

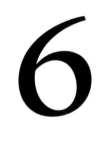

The purpose of this chapter is to develop the tools and skills set necessary to function effectively as a psychiatric nurse. Many of these skills are psychosocial interactive skills you will find transfer readily to any nursing setting as well as to the care of nonpsychiatric clients.

Reading Assignment

Please read Chapter 6, "Tools of Psychiatric Mental Health Nursing: Communication, Nursing Process, and the Nurse-Client Relationship," pages 97–111.

Key Terms

Write definitions for the following terms in your own words. Compare your definitions with those given in the text on page 98.

Defense Mechanisms _____

_____

Feedback _____

_____

Nonverbal Communication _____

_____

Orientation Phase _____

_____

Process Recording _____

_____

Termination Phase _____

_____

Therapeutic Communication _____

_____

Working Phase _____

_____

Exercises and Activities

1. Read the chapter opening box on page 97.

    a. What are some of the techniques you could use in establishing therapeutic relationships with clients?

    _____

    _____

    _____

    _____

    _____

    b. Identify the characteristics and differences between a therapeutic relationship and a personal relationship.

    _____

    _____

    _____

    _____

    _____

2. Review the Reflective Thinking box on page 100. List your most characteristic nonverbal gestures. Think about your smile, eye contact, hand movements, head nodding, and eyebrow movements.

    _____

    _____

    _____

    _____

    _____

3. Review the Reflective Thinking box on page 101. Under what circumstances would you consider "invading" a client's space, and why might this action be therapeutic in effect?

    _____

    _____

    _____

    _____

    _____

4. Study the "Summary of Therapeutic Communication Techniques" in Table 6-1 on page 102.

   a. Test yourself by covering one column at a time and filling in the missing content.

   b. Restate the meaning of each technique in your own words, including the purpose of each.

   _____

   _____

   _____

   _____

   _____

   _____

   _____

   _____

   _____

   _____

   _____

5. Review Table 6-2, "Common Defense Mechanisms," on page 104.

   a. Test yourself by covering one column at a time and filling in the missing content.

   b. In the following space, write an example for each of the defense mechanisms drawn from your own recent clinical experience. If you can't think of an example for one or more, ask your classmates or instructor to suggest an example.

   Symbolization

   _____

   Sublimation

   _____

   Suppression

   _____

   Regression

   _____

   Reaction formation

   _____

   Displacement

   _____

Introjection

_____

Rationalization

_____

Repression

_____

Projection

_____

Denial

_____

6. Read the Sample Process Recording in Table 6-3 on page 105.

a. Write a process recording drawn from a recent therapeutic interaction you have had with a client. Structure and analyze it according to the format in Table 6-3.

b. Critique your example. Is there anything you would have changed about the interaction?

_____

_____

_____

_____

_____

7. Review Figure 6-2, "Two Views of the Nursing Process," on page 106. Which view appeals more to you? Why?

_____

_____

_____

_____

_____

8. Review Table 6-4, "Elements of a Psychiatric History," on page 107. Note that the last item in the table is "Critical Decisions." Identify which of the preceding items in the table might contribute to the critical decisions and explain why.

_____

_____

_____

_____

_____

9. Review Table 6-5 on page 108 and think about the nursing process.

a. Explain the relationship between the elements of a psychiatric history (Table 6-4, page 107) and the nursing assessment.

_____

_____

_____

_____

_____

b. Write a nursing care plan for a client you have worked with recently.

c. Explain how you selected the nursing diagnosis in your plan. Would you need to have a therapeutic relationship with the client to accurately select the nursing diagnosis?

_____

_____

_____

_____

_____

d. How many of your evaluation/outcome statements represent long-term goals, and how many represent short-term goals? In relation to short-term and long-term goals, how much do the nursing and medical diagnoses seem to matter?

_____

_____

_____

_____

_____

e. What is the relationship between the planning step of the nursing process and the nursing theory you use to guide your practice?

_____

_____

_____

_____

_____

10. Review the "Five Aims of Intervention" box on page 109. Do the interventions in your care plan address all five aims? Why or why not?

_____

_____

_____

_____

_____

11. Read the case study of "Mrs. Rose M." on page 110.

a. In your own words, describe the phases of the nurse-client relationship as it is used in this case example.

_____

_____

_____

_____

_____

b. Which steps of the nursing process seem to correlate with each phase of the nurse-client interaction relationship?

_____

_____

_____

_____

_____

Self-Assessment Quiz

1. "Unconscious responses used by individuals to protect themselves from internal conflict and external stress" is a definition for which of the following terms? (page 98)

    a. Reflection

    b. Nonverbal communication

    c. Paralinguistic cues

    d. Defense mechanisms

2. All of the following are examples of nonverbal communication except (page 99)

    a. Physical space

    b. Action or kinetics

    c. Touch

    d. Listening

3. When a nursing student does a process recording, he/she should (page 104)

    a. tape record the conversation with the client and listen to it with the class.

    b. take notes during the conversation and take it to the supervisor for interpretation.

    c. write a nearly verbatim account of the conversation with the client, and interpret the techniques used and their effectiveness.

    d. write a report summarizing the conversation and use it to help formulate a nursing care plan.

4. Therapeutic communication techniques are best described as (page 102)

    a. Listening, silence, suggesting

    b. Broad openings, restating, informing

    c. Clarification, reflection, focusing, confronting

    d. All of the above

5. The nursing process incorporates which of the following elements? (page 105)

    a. Critical decision making, mental status examination, past medical history, chief complaint

    b. Identifying data, developmental and psychosocial history, outcomes, present illness history

    c. Mental status examination, planning interventions, nursing diagnosis, outcomes

    d. Assessment, nursing diagnosis, planning interventions, evaluation

6. Which of the following are examples of defense mechanisms? (page 103)

    a. Symbolization and denial

    b. Projection and displacement

    c. Regression and relating

    d. a and b

    e. a and c

7. All of the following are elements of a psychiatric history except (pages 105 and 107)

    a. Critical decisions

    b. Identifying data

    c. Impaired social interaction

    d. Mental status examination

8. Nursing diagnoses frequently seen in psychiatric nursing include all the following except (page 107)

    a. Risk for injury

    b. Depression

    c. Social isolation

    d. Post-trauma response

9. The nurse-client relationship includes which of the following phases? (page 109)

    a. Building trust phase, working phase, termination phase

    b. Orientation phase, promotion of strength phase, termination phase

    c. Orientation phase, working phase, termination phase

    d. All of the above

10. Which of the following concepts is most useful in dealing with psychiatric clients? (page 102)

    a. Verbal communication

    b. Therapeutic techniques

    c. Nonverbal communication

    d. Process recording

Cultural and Ethnic Considerations

7

The purpose of this chapter is to frame your thinking about the role of culture in mental illness and its treatment. This chapter encourages you to develop an awareness of your own culture and cultural identity, which can influence your feelings toward mental illness. You will consider the values and attitudes that act as prisms, coloring, refracting, distorting, and magnifying the cultural differences among individuals, as you encounter and treat people with mental illnesses.

Reading Assignment

Please read Chapter 7, "Cultural and Ethnic Considerations," pages 113–125.

Key Terms

Write definitions for the following terms in your own words. Compare your definitions with those given in the text on page 114.

Cultural Blindness _____

_____

Cultural Facilitator/Broker _____

_____

Culture _____

_____

Culture Shock _____

_____

Ethnicity _____

_____

Ethnocentrism_____

_____

Norms _____

_____

Stereotyping _____

_____

Values _____

_____

Exercises and Activities

1. Read the chapter opening box, "Know Your Own Culture," on page 113. Describe what you think another person might perceive about your cultural identity and cultural beliefs.

    _____

    _____

    _____

    _____

    _____

2. On page 117, the authors state that many nursing models of cultural assessment have been developed, citing Giger and Davidhizar and Andrews and Boyle as examples. They then explain the model they have used to organize this chapter. Have you thought about how you organize your cultural assessments? Develop a model you could use in your own practice, using the models cited for guidance.

    _____

    _____

    _____

    _____

    _____

3. Besides Western biomedical causation, name five agents that people worldwide believe cause mental illness. (page 117)

    _____

    _____

    _____

    _____

    _____

4. Read "Care Seeking and Acceptable Care" on pages 118–119.

    a. List the factors you can think of that people use to avoid or delay seeking general medical care.

_____

_____

_____

_____

_____

    b. List other factors that are roadblocks specific to seeking psychiatric/mental health care.

_____

_____

_____

_____

_____

    c. How would you counsel a person to overcome these particular reasons for not seeking psychiatric care?

_____

_____

_____

_____

_____

5. Seek out a person with a cultural background different from your own and engage the person in a casual conversation, making note of the following (pages 120–122):

    a. Eye contact

_____

_____

    b. Proxemics

_____

_____

   c. Touch

   _____

   _____

   d. Silence

   _____

   _____

   e. Social behavior

   _____

   _____

   f. Time orientation

   _____

   _____

6. Read the section on time orientation on page 122.

   a. Are you sequentially oriented or synchronically oriented? Why? Give an example.

   _____

   _____

   b. How would you determine which time orientation another person has?

   _____

   _____

   _____

   _____

   _____

c. What strategies would you use to interact effectively with a person whose time orientation is the opposite of your own?

_____

_____

_____

_____

_____

7. Write your personal definition of a "culturally competent mental health nurse." (page 124)

_____

_____

_____

_____

_____

8. As a cultural experiment, begin a conversation with a friend who has the same cultural background as you do. During the conversation, move in close to your friend, closer than you feel would be normal. (page 121)

a. How uncomfortable did this feel, and how long did it take for the discomfort to develop? What was your friend's reaction?

_____

_____

_____

_____

_____

b. Repeat the experiment, using silence as the variable. How long did your friend tolerate the silence? How uncomfortable do you feel in being silent during a conversation with your friend?

_____

_____

_____

_____

_____

   c. For people who may be depressed, anxious, or even psychotic, how much more uncomfortable do you think these violations of cultural norms would make them feel?

_____

_____

_____

_____

_____

9. Describe an incident in which you felt culturally out of place. Be sure to try to recreate your feelings. (page 122)

_____

_____

_____

_____

_____

10. You may already be aware that pain thresholds vary widely among cultural groups. Identify two other biological differences among cultural groups that have significance for care and treatment of mental illness. (pages 122–123)

_____

_____

_____

_____

_____

Self-Assessment Quiz

1. Norms are the learned beliefs about what is held as good or bad in a culture. (page 115)

   ❑ True

   ❑ False

2. The fair thing to do is to treat everybody the same and ignore differences in culture. (page 116)

   ❑ True

   ❑ False

3. CA + CK + CS + CE = CC. (page 116)

   ❑ True

   ❑ False

4. A client's punctuality is related to his or her time orientation. (page 122)

   ❑ True

   ❑ False

5. Just as a lack of appreciation for or knowledge of a client's cultural orientation can lead to insensitive and even harmful care, your failure to appreciate how well-integrated a minority group member may be into the mainstream North American culture could lead to the same. (page 124)

   ❑ True

   ❑ False

6. All of the following can be barriers to cultural sensitivity except (pages 115–118)

   a. cultural encounters.

   b. ethnocentrism.

   c. stereotyping.

   d. cultural blindness.

7. Which of the following is a sure sign of mental illness? (page 118)

   a. Abnormal behavior

   b. Inappropriate behavior

   c. Silence

   d. Rudeness

   e. None of the above

8. Mental illness can be attributed to (page 118)

   a. sorcery.

   b. violating taboos.

   c. environmental imbalances.

   d. laziness.

9. A cultural facilitator or broker can do all of the following except (page 120)

    a. Understand the health beliefs of the client's culture

    b. Arrange to pay for health care

    c. Interpret in the client's native language

    d. Explain the health care system to the client

10. The communication problem a nurse can most easily solve is (page 124)

    a. unappreciated cultural considerations.

    b. altered thought processes.

    c. fear or mistrust.

    d. age and sex differences.

Epidemiology of Mental Health and Illness

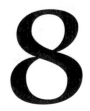

The purpose of this chapter is to establish the incidence and prevalence of mental illness, to explain how mental illnesses are categorized and diagnosed, and to suggest research areas that need to be explored in future studies.

Reading Assignment

Please read Chapter 8, "Epidemiology of Mental Health and Illness," pages 127–137.

Key Terms

Write definitions for the following terms in your own words. Compare your definitions with those given in the text on page 128.

Blinded Clinical Trial _____

_____

Case-Control Study _____

_____

Cohort Study _____

_____

Control Group _____

_____

Controlled Clinical Trial _____

_____

Descriptive Study _____

_____

Double-Blinded Trial _____

_____

Endemic _____

_____

Epidemic _____

_____

Epidemiology _____

_____

Experimental Group _____

_____

Incidence _____

_____

Interrater Agreement _____

_____

Interrater Reliability _____

_____

Intrarater Reliability _____

_____

Longitudinal Study _____

_____

Meta-analysis _____

_____

Placebo _____

_____

Prevalence _____

_____

Quasi-Experimental Study _____

_____

Reliability _____

_____

Risk Factors _____

_____

Validity _____

_____

Exercises and Activities

1. Read the chapter opening box on page 127. What role do you feel nurses should play in the development of public health policy?

    _____

    _____

    _____

    _____

    _____

2. In your own words, state as many goals of epidemiology as you can. (pages 129–130)

_____

_____

_____

_____

_____

3. Explain the difference between a blinded and a double-blinded controlled clinical trial. (page 129)

_____

_____

_____

_____

_____

4. Explain the difference between incidence and prevalence. (page 130)

_____

_____

_____

_____

_____

5. Explain the difference between descriptive and quasi-experimental studies and state the significance of the difference. (page 130)

_____

_____

_____

_____

_____

6. Take the timeline you created in Chapter 2 (Exercise and Activity #5) and superimpose the various revisions of the DSM on it. (page 131)

    a. What correlations emerge?

    _____

    _____

    _____

    _____

    _____

    b. Add the major landmark studies referenced in this chapter, including the Epidemiologic Catchment Area Study.

7. In your own words, state the purposes of the DSM and its use in psychiatric nursing. (pages 131–132)

    _____

    _____

    _____

    _____

    _____

8. Stigmatization is one of the major reasons why people with mental illnesses often avoid seeking treatment. Labeling contributes to stigmatizing. What devices do the authors of this textbook use to avoid labeling? Read the Reflective Thinking box on page 131. What strategies can you incorporate into your own clinical practice to avoid labeling and unnecessary stigmatizing?

    _____

    _____

    _____

    _____

    _____

9. Refer to the DSM-IV-TR Classification in Appendix C on pages 808–816 for the currently accepted labels for the entire range of psychiatric disorders.

   a. Do any of these labels surprise you? Did this exercise enhance your understanding of the range of disorders classified as psychiatric disorders? Did this exercise help you organize mental disorders better in your mind?

   _____

   _____

   _____

   _____

   _____

   b. Review the descriptions of mood disorders, schizophrenia, substance abuse disorders, and anxiety disorders on page 132. List the major diagnostic criteria for each of these groups of disorders.

   Mood disorders

   _____

   _____

   _____

   _____

   _____

   Schizophrenia

   _____

   _____

   _____

   _____

   _____

   Substance abuse disorders

   _____

   _____

   _____

   _____

   _____

Anxiety disorders

_____

_____

_____

_____

____._____

c. How difficult do you think it would be to diagnose someone with one of these disorders?

_____

_____

_____

_____

_____

10. What were the significant findings of the three early epidemiological studies in Stirling County, Nova Scotia; Manhattan; and Baltimore? (pages 132–133)

_____

_____

_____

_____

_____

11. Review the questions on page 133 raised by the Carter Commission. For which of these questions was the resulting Epidemiologic Catchment Area (ECA) Study able to provide some answers?

_____

_____

_____

_____

_____

12. Which results of the ECA Study surprised you the most? (page 134)

_____

_____

_____

_____

_____

13. What is the tip-of-the-iceberg phenomenon? (pages 134–135)

_____

_____

_____

_____

_____

14. Summarize the main finding of the National Comorbidity Study (NCS). How would you compare the comorbidity of psychiatric disorders with that of medical-surgical disorders?

_____

_____

_____

_____

_____

Self-Assessment Quiz

1. Early studies of the incidence and prevalence of mental illness showed that mental illness is widespread in the general population. (pages 132–133)

   ❑ True

   ❑ False

2. Mental illnesses tend to be endemic rather than epidemic. (page 129)

   ❑ True

   ❑ False

3. Risk factors can be clues to the causes of diseases. (page 129)

   ❑ True

   ❑ False

4. Both descriptive and quasi-experimental studies can be longitudinal. (page 130)

   ❑ True

   ❑ False

5. Only psychiatrists can use the DSM to diagnose clients. (page 131)

   ❑ True

   ❑ False

6. The Carter Commission wanted answers to which of the following questions? (page 133)

   a. How much would a massive mental health study cost?

   b. Should Medicare cover major mental disorders?

   c. What are the causes of mental illness?

   d. Does poverty contribute to the severity of mental illness?

   e. b and c

   f. c and d

7. Which of the following is *not* a result of choosing the wrong sample size for a study? (pages 133–134)

   a. People won't have confidence in the results if it is too small.

   b. The results won't be valid if it is too small.

   c. The results will be confusing if it is too big.

   d. A sample too large would be a waste of money.

8. The tip-of-the-iceberg phenomenon means that (pages 134–135)

   a. many people have symptoms but only a few seek help.

   b. only a small number of mentally ill people are severely mentally ill.

   c. life is frought with hidden perils.

   d. there are not enough resources to care for everyone with mental illness.

9. According to the NCS, what is the comorbidity? (page 136)

    a. 10%

    b. 90%

    c. 70%

    d. 50%

10. Cognitive impairment is

    a. not a DSM diagnosis.

    b. more prevalent among older people.

    c. a major, underrecognized public health problem.

    d. All of the above

Ethical and Legal Bases for Care

9

Τhe purpose of this chapter is to provide you with the ethical theories and legal information you need to guide your practice. Conducting nursing care in a manner that conforms to the law and adheres to the highest ethical standards protects you from lawsuits and protects your clients from abuse, manipulation, and shoddy health care. In the area of mental health practice, there are many unique ethical issues and highly specific laws that apply to the conduct of psychiatric care.

Reading Assignment

Please read Chapter 9, "Ethical and Legal Bases for Care," pages 139–154.

Key Terms

Write definitions for the following terms in your own words. Compare your definitions with those given in the text on pages 140–141.

Abandonment _____

_____

Autonomy _____

_____

Beneficence _____

_____

Civil Commitment _____

_____

Code of Ethics _____

_____

Competency to Stand Trial _____

_____

Conservator _____

_____

Deontology _____

_____

Emergency Hospitalization _____

_____

Ethics _____

_____

Fidelity _____

_____

Incompetence _____

_____

Justice _____

_____

Least Restrictive Alternative _____

_____

Malpractice _____

_____

M'Naghten Test _____

_____

Negligence _____

_____

Nonmaleficence _____

_____

Normative Ethics _____

_____

Physical Restraint _____

_____

Probate Proceedings _____

_____

Seclusion _____

_____

Tarasoff Duty to Warn _____

_____

Utilitarianism _____

_____

Exercises and Activities

1. Read the chapter opening box on page 139.

   a. Do you feel in control when you have a client under your care? List ways in which you have power or control over that client.

   _____

   _____

   _____

   _____

   _____

   b. Do you conduct your professional practice in a manner deserving of the trust the public has in the nursing profession? List some of the "rules" you have that guide your practice.

   _____

   _____

   _____

   _____

   _____

2. Read the Reflective Thinking box on page 142.

   a. Do you think Harold needs health care help? What would you do to try to help him?

   _____

   _____

   _____

   _____

   _____

   b. Would you enlist the support of any other health care professionals to help him?

   _____

   _____

   _____

   _____

   _____

c.   Do you believe health care should be mandated for Harold? Explain why or why not.

_____

_____

_____

_____

_____

d.   If your decision making were guided by ethical theory alone, what action would you take based on the following ethical theories?

Utilitarianism

_____

_____

_____

_____

_____

Autonomy

_____

_____

_____

_____

_____

Beneficence

_____

_____

_____

_____

_____

Nonmaleficence

_____

_____

_____

_____

_____

3. Write your response to the authors' observation that "laws attempt to provide for the public good and public safety, but rarely do the laws offer comprehensive solutions to social problems . . ." (page 145).

_____

_____

_____

_____

_____

4. Laws often regulate conflicting interests. Match the conflicting rights in the two columns by drawing lines between them. (pages 145–149)

Right to treatment	Right to safety
Right to an orderly treatment environment	Right of many against few
	Right to refuse treatment
Right to informed consent	Right not to be restrained or secluded
Right of free speech	
Right to privacy	Right to refuse consent
Right to keep personal items	Right to be informed of threats

5. What does the American Psychological Association's Mental Health Patient's Bill of Rights cover? What other rights, if any, do you think mental health patients should have?

_____

_____

_____

_____

_____

6. Mark David Chapman shot and killed John Lennon. Refusing the insanity defense, he pleaded guilty and received a sentence of 20 years to life. John Hinckley shot and wounded then-President Ronald Reagan in an effort to impress actress Jody Foster. He was found guilty by reason of insanity. The American poet Ezra Pound made radio broadcasts during World War II in support of Italian dictator Benito Mussolini and was charged with treason. He was kept in a psychiatric hospital for years before charges were dropped and he was allowed to spend his remaining years in Italy. Juries rejected the insanity defense for serial killers Jeffrey Dahmer, John Wayne Gacy, and David "Son of Sam" Berkowitz (who later admitted he made up his story of receiving messages to kill from barking dogs). (page 147)

a. What is the rule of law that provides for the insanity defense?

_____

_____

_____

_____

_____

b. What is your opinion of the "insanity defense"?

_____

_____

_____

_____

_____

c. Could you provide quality nursing care for a client who had committed a crime but had been declared not guilty by reason of insanity?

_____

_____

_____

_____

_____

d. Ethically and/or legally, would you be under any obligation to provide treatment to that client?

_____

_____

_____

_____

_____

7. A widely cited New York case, *Rivers v. Katz* (1986), provides guidelines to follow when clients can be given medication against their will. (page 148)

a. State the four guidelines established by the court.

_____

_____

_____

_____

_____

b. Are these guidelines used in your state? If not, are any other guidelines in place?

_____

_____

_____

_____

_____

8. Consider the Reflective Thinking box on informed consent, regarding Mrs. Roebuck, on page 150.

a. Is there a clear-cut consent to treatment from Mrs. Roebuck? Why or why not?

_____

_____

_____

_____

_____

b. If you were the nurse caring for Mrs. Roebuck, what would you do to make yourself feel more comfortable that the informed consent issue was handled properly?

_____

_____

_____

_____

_____

9. What elements are necessary and desirable in obtaining informed consent? (pages 149–150)

_____

_____

_____

_____

_____

10. In dealing with clients who may have altered thought processes, extreme preoccupation, a flat affect, or regressed behavior, obtaining informed consent for treatment becomes a gray area of judgment for the clinician. (pages 150–151)

a. How would you decide whether a client had the capacity to provide informed consent?

_____

_____

_____

_____

_____

b. Are there any special measures you could take to demonstrate that informed consent was obtained in a careful, responsible manner?

_____

_____

_____

_____

_____

11. Numerous legal and ethical obligations apply to the psychiatric mental health nurse. Although laws vary from state to state, some well-established guidelines are virtually universal. (pages 150–153)

    a. When a clinician becomes aware that a client has made a specific threat of bodily harm against a specific individual, what is the clinician's responsibility?

_____

_____

_____

_____

_____

    b. When a clinician is informed that child abuse is taking place, what is the clinician's duty?

_____

_____

_____

_____

_____

    c. When clinicians discontinue professional practice, what is their obligation to their clients?

_____

_____

_____

_____

_____

    d. When is it appropriate for a clinician to have a sexual relationship with a client or former client?

_____

_____

_____

_____

_____

e. When is it appropriate to release confidential information about a client?

_____

_____

_____

_____

_____

f. When is it appropriate to violate the civil rights of a client?

_____

_____

_____

_____

_____

Self-Assessment Quiz

1. Sedating a client with neuroleptic medication is a way of getting around troublesome laws regulating physical restraint. (page 148)

   ❑ True

   ❑ False

2. Physical restraint or seclusion may be appropriate for clients who are a danger to themselves or others if these are the least restrictive alternatives. (page 151)

   ❑ True

   ❑ False

3. The nurse's duty to protect a client's privacy and confidentiality takes precedence over the duty to warn a specific individual of a violent threat a client has made toward the individual. (page 151)

   ❑ True

   ❑ False

4. Abandonment is a form of negligence that could lead to a malpractice suit. (page 151)

   ❑ True

   ❑ False

5. Clients who are dangerous to themselves or others can usually be hospitalized against their will on an emergency basis for a short period of two to three days as an extension of local police powers. (page 152)

   ❑ True

   ❑ False

6. All of the following are legitimate ethical theories used to guide ethical decision making in the health care sector except (pages 142–143)

   a. Situational ethics

   b. Utilitarianism

   c. Justice

   d. Autonomy

7. Clients have all of the following rights except (pages 145–149)

   a. Civil rights

   b. Right to keep personal items

   c. Right to choose the nurse assigned to them

   d. Right to informed consent

8. All of the following are the usual and/or prudent elements of informed consent except (pages 146–147)

   a. All risks associated with the treatment

   b. Description, length, and cost of treatment

   c. Clinician's note in client record and consent signed by client

   d. Most significant risks associated with treatment

9. For a client to be involuntarily committed to a psychiatric facility, a court has to hear compelling evidence of any of the following except (page 149)

   a. Dangerous to self

   b. Dangerous to others

   c. Insulting or vulgar to judge

   d. Unable to care for basic needs

10. The nurse has the right to release confidential information about a client in all but one of the following situations. (page 146)

    a. The client signs a release.

    b. The client is a celebrity and the request comes from the media.

    c. An officer of the court has a signed court order.

    d. Another health professional is directly involved in the care of the client.

The Client Undergoing Crisis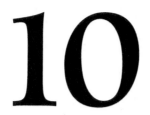

The purpose of this chapter is to help you understand the stages of a crisis, evaluate coping mechanisms, and implement interventions that may lessen the impact of a crisis.

Reading Assignment

Please read Chapter 10, "The Client Undergoing Crisis," pages 157–159.

Key Terms

Write definitions for the following terms in your own words. Compare your definitions with those given in the text on page 159.

Adaptive Energy_____

_____

Adaptive Potential Assessment Model _____

_____

Arousal_____

_____

Community Crisis _____

_____

Conservative-Withdrawal State _____

_____

Crisis_____

_____

Cultural Crisis_____

_____

Culture Shock _____

_____

Equilibrium _____

_____

Fight-Flight Response _____

_____

General Adaptation Syndrome_____

_____

Impoverishment _____

_____

Maturational Crisis _____

_____

Psychological Development _____

_____

Situational Crisis_____

_____

Stress _____

_____

Exercises and Activities

1. Pick a crisis from your own experience and use it as a focal point throughout this chapter. (pages 159–170)

    a. Describe the crisis you've chosen. What type of crisis is it?

    _____

    _____

    _____

    _____

    _____

    b. What support systems, if any, did you use in managing your crisis?

    _____

    _____

    _____

    _____

    _____

c. What coping skills did you use to reduce your anxiety?

_____

_____

_____

_____

_____

d. What features of your personality did you use to help you cope with this crisis?

_____

_____

_____

_____

_____

e. What nursing theory would you suggest for a nurse caring for you in this crisis?

_____

_____

_____

_____

_____

2. Name and differentiate the four types of crises, noting their distinguishing characteristics. (page 161)

_____

_____

_____

_____

_____

3. What are Caplan's four phases of a crisis? (page 161)

_____

_____

_____

_____

_____

  a. What can an individual do to escape from an escalating crisis?

  _____

  _____

  _____

  _____

  _____

  b. What possible outcomes can individuals experience if they are not able to prevent the escalation of a crisis?

  _____

  _____

  _____

  _____

4. What is the relationship between developmental stages and stress? Describe the ways people of different ages are likely to respond to stress.

_____

_____

_____

_____

_____

5. What are the phases of Selye's General Adaptation Syndrome? Relate these phases to the personal crisis you identified above. What specific behaviors did you exhibit during the various phases of your crisis? (page 162)

_____

_____

_____

_____

_____

6. When should you evaluate a client in crisis for suicide risk? (page 171)

_____

_____

_____

_____

_____

7. List nursing diagnoses that often apply to people in crises. (page 171)

_____

_____

_____

_____

_____

8. Have you ever experienced culture shock? List the nursing diagnoses that might have applied to this experience. (page 170)

_____

_____

_____

_____

_____

9. What is the main intent of the crisis intervention model? (page 173)

_____

_____

_____

_____

_____

Self-Assessment Quiz

1. It is important to include time frames in outcome statements, because time frames can indicate how well a client is managing a crisis. (page 172)

   ❑ True

   ❑ False

2. Crisis intervention skills are more important on an inpatient unit than in the community. (page 174)

   ❑ True

   ❑ False

3. Cultural crisis and culture shock are the same thing. (page 170)

   ❑ True

   ❑ False

4. A hurricane can be both a situational and a community crisis. (page 161)

   ❑ True

   ❑ False

5. Crisis, by definition, calls for adaptation. (page 159)

   ❑ True

   ❑ False

6. All of the following are typical responses to stress except (page 162)

    a. Adaptation

    b. Fight-flight

    c. Attraction-repulsion

    d. Conservative-withdrawal

7. Major stressors in today's society include (page 165)

    a. weekends.

    b. television.

    c. drug addiction.

    d. church or temple.

8. The goal of adaptation can be characterized by all the following terms except (page 166)

    a. Balance

    b. Equilibrium

    c. Homeostasis

    d. Arousal

9. All of the following can be effective nursing strategies for a client in crisis except (page 173)

    a. Unconditional caring

    b. Allowing for grieving

    c. Pointing out how lucky the client is in other areas of life

    d. Fostering communication about crisis

10. Which nursing diagnosis would have little application to a client in crisis? (page 171)

    a. Anxiety

    b. Chronic low self-esteem

    c. Dysfunctional grieving

    d. Fear

The Client Experiencing Anxiety

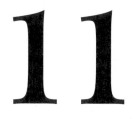

The purpose of this chapter is to gain an understanding of when anxiety, which is to some extent a normal part of our everyday lives, becomes problematical and pathological. How can the nurse recognize harmful anxiety, and what nursing care is then appropriate?

Reading Assignment

Please read Chapter 11, "The Client Experiencing Anxiety," pages 181–215

Key Terms

Write definitions for the following terms in your own words. Compare your definitions with those given in the text on page 183.

Adversity _____

_____

Agoraphobia _____

_____

Anxiety _____

_____

Cognitive-Behavior Therapy _____

_____

Compulsion _____

_____

Fear _____

_____

Generalized Anxiety Disorder _____

_____

Obsession _____

_____

Panic Disorder _____

_____

Phobia _____

_____

Positron Emission Tomography (PET) _____

_____

Post-Traumatic Stress Disorder _____

_____

Trait Anxiety _____

_____

Exercises and Activities

1. Review the Nursing Tip on page 184.

    a. What is the critical difference between fear and anxiety?

    _____

    _____

    _____

    _____

    _____

    b. How is your personal response to fear different from your personal response to anxiety?

    _____

    _____

    _____

    _____

    _____

    c. Can you think of any positive outcomes of fear and anxiety?

    _____

    _____

    _____

    _____

    _____

2. What are the physiological manifestations of fear and anxiety? Do the two feelings differ in terms of physiological response? (pages 185–186)

_____

_____

_____

_____

_____

3. What do philosophers and writers mean when they characterize the twentieth century as the "age of anxiety"? (pages 186, 187)

_____

_____

_____

_____

_____

4. Review Table 11-1, "Stages of Anxiety," on page 187.

   a. What are the differences among the stages?

   _____

   _____

   _____

   _____

   _____

   b. Give an example of each stage.

   _____

   _____

   _____

   _____

   _____

5. Review Table 11-2, "Summary of Major Anxiety Disorders," on page 188. Test your knowledge by covering one column at a time and verbalizing the hidden information.

6. What are the symptoms of a panic disorder? (pages 188–189)

   _____

   _____

   _____

   _____

   _____

7. Do you know anyone who experiences a fear of flying? What does this fear have in common with all other phobias? What are the treatment options?

   _____

   _____

   _____

   _____

   _____

8. Read the Nursing Tip on page 193. How would you determine if a client in an Emergency Department were experiencing Social Anxiety Disroder? What kind of therapeutic communication strategies would you employ with such an individual?

   _____

   _____

   _____

   _____

   _____

9. Review the model for anxiety in Figure 11-1 on page 200.

   a. What is the difference between adversity and trait anxiety?

   _____

   _____

   _____

   _____

   _____

    b. How would you use this model in your practice?

_____

_____

_____

_____

_____

    c. Do you experience trait anxiety? If not, how do you know? If so, how pronounced is your trait?

_____

_____

_____

_____

_____

10. Think about a client experiencing anxiety over a particular event, such as taking a test. (page 188)

    a. What symptoms would the client be experiencing?

_____

_____

_____

_____

    b. What behavioral counseling would you offer the client? (Think about humor, guided imagery, relaxation techniques, related insights, and other modalities you are familiar with.)

_____

_____

_____

_____

_____

11. Many people can point to examples of obsessive or compulsive behavior in their own lives without being diagnosed as having Obsessive-Compulsive Disorder. When do simple repetitive or irresistible behaviors become diagnosable as a disorder? (pages 194–195)

_____

_____

_____

_____

_____

12. Emil F. appears in the Emergency Department where you work shortly after a gunshot incident in the school where he teaches eighth grade science. Although no one was seriously injured, the incident took place in the classroom next to where Emil was teaching. He is clasping his hands together and he appears frightened and teary. He states that he has been hyperventilating and cannot seem to regain his composure. He says he is not sure he will be able to return to work.

    a. In all likelihood, what is Mr. F. suffering from?

    _____

    _____

    _____

    _____

    b. What nursing diagnosis would you assess for?

    _____

    _____

    _____

    _____

    c. What nursing interventions would you perform? What outcomes would be optimal for each intervention?

    _____

    _____

    _____

    _____

    _____

Self-Assessment Quiz

1. Generalized Anxiety Disorder is a "diagnosis of exclusion." (page 187)
   - ❑ True
   - ❑ False

2. Clients in panic attacks consider suicide more often than clients with any other psychiatric disorder. (page 189)
   - ❑ True
   - ❑ False

3. Most phobias begin in early childhood. (page 192)
   - ❑ True
   - ❑ False

4. The physiological causes of anxiety have been well understood for almost one hundred years. (page 185)
   - ❑ True
   - ❑ False

5. Moderate to severe anxiety always profoundly interferes with an individual's ability to function normally in life. (page 187)
   - ❑ True
   - ❑ False

6. The percentage of the population afflicted with phobias is (page 192)
   - a. 2%.
   - b. 5%.
   - c. 10%.
   - d. 50%.

7. All of the following are standard treatments for anxiety except (pages 200–202)

    a. Psychotherapy

    b. Pharmacotherapy

    c. Behavioral therapy

    d. Isolation therapy

8. All of the following are legitimate nursing responses to a client with anxiety except (pages 204–206)

    a. Identifying the type of anxiety from which the client is suffering

    b. Offering cognitive-behavioral therapy

    c. Telling the client to "snap out of it" or "laugh it off"

    d. Trying to understand the client's subjective experience of anxiety

9. All of the following may contribute to the development of Post-Traumatic Stress Disorder except (page 197)

    a. Degree of victim's imagination

    b. Extreme violence of precipitating event

    c. Poor pre-trauma mental health

    d. Lack of post-trauma support systems

10. Positron emission tomography (PET) images show the following changes when clients with anxiety disorders are confronted with anxiety-producing stimuli (page 185)

    a. No changes

    b. Changes in electrical thresholds

    c. Changes in blood flow

    d. Structural changes

The Client Experiencing Schizophrenia

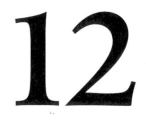

The purpose of Chapter 12 is to present a vivid clinical picture of the client experiencing schizophrenia. At the same time, the disease is demystified, with a discussion of the range of the illness, its possible causes, clinical course, treatment, and therapeutic nursing care.

Reading Assignment

Please read Chapter 12, "The Client Experiencing Schizophrenia," pages 217–243.

Key Terms

Write definitions for the following terms in your own words. Compare your definitions with those in the text on page 219.

Akathisia _____

_____

Akinesia _____

_____

Alogia _____

_____

Anhedonia _____

_____

Avolition _____

_____

Catatonia _____

_____

Delusion _____

_____

Derailment _____

_____

Dystonia _____

_____

Flattened Affect _____

_____

Grandiose Delusion _____

Hallucination _____

_____

Incoherence _____

_____

Neologistic Word _____

_____

Persecutory Delusion _____

_____

Psychotic _____

_____

Referential Delusion _____

_____

Schizophrenia _____

_____

Tangentiality _____

_____

Tardive Dyskinesia _____

_____

Word Salad _____

_____

Exercises and Activities

1. Review the chapter opening box on page 217.

    a. Have you thought about what it would be like to care for someone who has a thought disorder?

    _____

    b. How do you plan to prepare yourself for this work?

    _____

    _____

    _____

    _____

    _____

2. Review the "Dispelling Common Myths about Schizophrenia" box on page 219.

    a. Did you believe any of these myths? Write a statement that reflects your corrected thinking.

    _____

    _____

    _____

    _____

    _____

    b. Go to the Online Companion for Frisch and Frisch's *Psychiatric Mental Health Nursing* located at http://www.DelmarNursing.com. Read the online chapter on Multiple Personality Disorder. Did reading this chapter help sharpen your understanding of schizophrenia?

    _____

    _____

    _____

    _____

    _____

3. Read the Anonymous Autobiography on pages 219 and 220.

    a. Were you surprised that the author was functioning in a role similar to yours? How much more difficult would your role as a student be if you had schizophrenia?

    _____

    _____

    _____

    _____

    _____

    b. Why do you think this author kept her anonymity?

    _____

    _____

    _____

    _____

    _____

4. Read the three self-reports of delusions on pages 222 and 223.

   a. Write as many adjectives as come to mind as you read these descriptions. What kind of picture emerges in your mind?

   _____

   _____

   _____

   _____

   _____

   b. How would you respond to a client who reported these delusions to you? What strategies might you use to respond therapeutically?

   _____

   _____

   _____

   _____

   _____

5. Compare and contrast delusions with hallucinations. (pages 223–225)

   _____

   _____

   _____

   _____

   _____

6. Compare and contrast the positive symptoms of schizophrenia with the negative symptoms of schizophrenia. (pages 223–225)

   _____

   _____

   _____

   _____

   _____

7. The authors write on page 223, ". . . some writers and psychiatrists have portrayed persons with schizophrenia as individualistic heroes in a society that celebrates conformity and materialistic values . . . " What is your response to this statement?

    _____

    _____

    _____

    _____

    _____

8. Examine the PET brain images on page 224. What would you conclude about the brain's ability to differentiate between a hallucination brought about as a result of a psychotic state and the actual experience of the image being hallucinated?

    _____

    _____

    _____

    _____

    _____

9. Review Figure 12-1, "Genetic risk for developing schizophrenia," on page 229.

    a. What is the risk in the general population of developing schizophrenia?

    _____

    b. According to this figure, what percentage of people with schizophrenia had a parent who had schizophrenia?

    _____

10. State in your own words the current scientific understanding of the cause of schizophrenia. How would you explain to the parent of a teenager recently diagnosed with schizophrenia what the cause is likely to be? (pages 229–230)

    _____

    _____

    _____

    _____

    _____

11.   Describe the two major approaches to the treatment of schizophrenia. (pages 230–235)

_____

_____

_____

_____

_____

12.   Read the Nursing Tip on page 231.

   a.   What nursing needs do families of clients with schizophrenia have?

_____

_____

_____

_____

_____

   b.   What kind of a therapeutic program would you design for families of clients with schizophrenia?

_____

_____

_____

_____

_____

13.   Read the Reflective Thinking box on page 232.

   a.   Make a list of pros and cons on the issue of deinstitutionalization.

_____

_____

_____

_____

_____

b. Explain why you think a policy of deinstitutionalization was pursued in the 1970s.

_____

_____

_____

_____

_____

14. Read the discussion of pharmacological treatment of schizophrenia on pages 233–235.

a. Compare and contrast the positives and the negatives associated with treatment of schizophrenia with neuroleptic drugs.

_____

_____

_____

_____

_____

b. Compare atypical neuroleptics with older neuroleptics.

_____

_____

_____

_____

_____

15. Read the Case Study about "Gary" on page 239. Then, review Table 12-1, "Symptoms Experienced with Schizophrenia and Associated Nursing Diagnoses," on page 229, and the Nursing Diagnosis Section on page 237.

a. Which of these symptoms does Gary seem to suffer?

_____

_____

_____

_____

_____

b. Write two additional nursing diagnosis statements for Gary, using the information in the Case Study.

_____

_____

_____

_____

_____

16. Classify the following symptoms of schizophrenia according to whether they are positive (P) symptoms or negative (N) symptoms (pages 220–226):

a. _____Delusions

b. _____Lack of motivation

c. _____Flat affect

d. _____Hallucinations

e. _____Paranoia

f. _____Word salad

g. _____Poor hygiene or grooming

h. _____Poverty of speech

i. _____Poor eye contact

j. _____Grandiose or all-powerful thoughts

k. _____Inability to function

Learning Tip: Positive symptoms are traits "added" to the normal personality, aspects most people don't have, like delusions. Negative symptoms are traits "deleted" from the normal personality, deficits most people don't have, like inability to function.

17. Compare and contrast the acute and rehabilitative phases of schizophrenia in terms of (page 237):

a. Treatment goals

_____

_____

_____

_____

_____

b. Nurse's role

_____

_____

_____

_____

_____

Self-Assessment Quiz

1. Schizophrenia is an illness diagnosed in early childhood, usually between the ages of 1 and 6. (page 226)

    ❑   True

    ❑   False

2. Schizophrenia is a costly illness, both financially and medically. (page 227)

    ❑   True

    ❑   False

3. Neuroleptic medication has been helpful to clients with schizophrenia since 1952. (page 233)

    ❑   True

    ❑   False

4. Neuroleptic medication can cause severe, nonreversible side effects. (page 233)

    ❑   True

    ❑   False

5. Tardive dyskinesia is one of the mild, reversible side effects of neuroleptic medication. (page 234)

    ❑   True

    ❑   False

6. Dystonia is a side effect of neuroleptic medication which is characterized by painful muscle spasms that can last from a few seconds to a few days. (page 233)

   ❑ True

   ❑ False

7. Clients with schizophrenia pose a low risk for suicide. (page 227)

   ❑ True

   ❑ False

8. The psychoanalytic theory of schizophrenia was based on Jean Piaget's work. (page 228)

   ❑ True

   ❑ False

9. Delusions, hallucinations, and grandiosity are all negative symptoms of schizophrenia. (pages 222–223)

   ❑ True

   ❑ False

10. Anhedonia means the loss of ability to enjoy a normally pleasurable activity. (page 219)

    ❑ True

    ❑ False

11. The brain differences in clients with schizophrenia have been divided into two categories, anatomical and functional; an enlarged ventricle would be in the anatomical category. (pages 229–230)

    ❑ True

    ❑ False

12. Akathisia is a side effect of neuroleptic medication characterized by a poverty of movement. (page 234)

    ❑ True

    ❑ False

13. Clozapine is a new atypical neuroleptic with no major side effects. (page 234)

    ❏ True

    ❏ False

14. Most psychiatric nurses are able to form a therapeutic relationship with a client who is in the acute phase of schizophrenia. (page 236)

    ❏ True

    ❏ False

15. The nurse should try to persuade clients with schizophrenia that they are not hearing voices or seeing things that aren't there. (page 236)

    ❏ True

    ❏ False

16. The main goal of treatment for a client in the acute phase of schizophrenia is to control the symptoms. (page 238)

    ❏ True

    ❏ False

17. The MRI images of brains from clients with schizophrenia have which of the following differences from brains of clients without schizophrenia? (page 229)

    a. The hippocampus is much larger in clients with schizophrenia.

    b. The ventricles are larger in the clients with schizophrenia.

    c. The hippocampus is much smaller in clients with schizophrenia.

    d. b and c

18. Which two of the following theories have never been seriously considered as the cause of schizophrenia? (pages 228–230)

    a. Genetics

    b. Cause will never be known

    c. Lead poisoning

    d. Inadequate maternal nurturing

    e. Dopamine hypothesis

    f. Phases of the moon

    g. Organic causes

19. Which of the following nursing diagnoses is most likely associated with the rehabilitative phase of schizophrenia? (page 237)

    a. Altered sensory perception

    b. Impaired verbal communication

    c. Ineffective management of therapeutic regimen

    d. Sleep pattern disturbance

20. Which of the following nursing interventions would not be appropriate for managing a client in the rehabilitative phase of schizophrenia? (page 238)

    a. Monitor compliance with medication regime

    b. Promote social isolation

    c. Urge client to make a daily schedule and stick with it

    d. Involve family members in the treatment program

The Client Experiencing Depression

13

The purpose of this chapter is to understand the illness of depression in its various forms. Ups, downs, and mood changes are a normal part of life. How dreary and unfulfilling life would be if everyone were cheerful and upbeat all the time! Depressive disorders occur when the downswings in mood are deep, unrelenting, and dysfunctional. Learning to recognize and respond to depression is an essential skill for nurses, because depression is a pervasive and devastating illness frequently seen in clients hospitalized for other medical reasons.

Reading Assignment

Please read Chapter 13, "The Client Experiencing Depression," pages 245–275.

Key Terms

Write definitions for the following terms in your own words. Compare your definitions with those given in the text on page 247.

Bipolar Depression _____

_____

Brief Dynamic Therapy _____

_____

Chronic Grief _____

_____

Cognitive Therapy _____

_____

Delayed Grief _____

_____

Depression _____

_____

Ego _____

_____

Exaggerated Grief _____

_____

Grief _____

_____

Marital Therapy _____

_____

Masked Grief _____

_____

Mood Disorder _____

_____

Mood Episode _____

_____

Nurse Agency _____

_____

Self-Care Agency _____

_____

Superego _____

_____

Supportive-Educative Role _____

_____

Unipolar Depression _____

_____

Exercises and Activities

1. Much of the important content of this chapter has to do with diagnosing depression and differentiating it from the normal ups and downs of daily experience.

   a. Describe the difference between a Minor Depressive Disorder and a Major Depressive Disorder.

   _____

   _____

   _____

   _____

   _____

b. Describe the difference between a Major Depressive Episode and a Major Depressive Disorder.

_____

_____

_____

_____

_____

c. What are the major symptoms of depression?

_____

_____

_____

_____

_____

d. What factors and symptoms must be present for there to be a diagnosis of Major Depressive Disorder?

_____

_____

_____

_____

_____

e. Describe the differences between Major Depressive Disorder and Dysthymic Disorder.

_____

_____

_____

_____

_____

f.   Describe the differences between depression and grief.

_____

_____

_____

_____

_____

2.   Almost 15% of all hospitalized clients meet the criteria for Major Depressive Disorder. What may be misleading or complicating about this statistic? (pages 249–251)

_____

_____

_____

_____

_____

3.   List the risk factors for depression. (page 254)

_____

_____

_____

_____

_____

4.   List the theories of depression. (pages 257–258)

_____

_____

_____

_____

_____

a. To which theory do you most subscribe, and why?

_____

_____

_____

_____

_____

b. Which other theories merit serious evaluation, in your view, and why?

_____

_____

_____

_____

_____

5. Describe the stages of bereavement. (pages 254–257)

_____

_____

_____

_____

_____

6. Have you experienced the death of a loved one in your life?

a. Describe your grief response, relating it to the stages you identified previously.

_____

_____

_____

_____

_____

b. How would you evaluate successful grieving in yourself or in a client you are treating?

_____

_____

_____

_____

_____

7. Identify the four types of dysfunctional grieving, and describe their unique characteristics. (page 256)

_____

_____

_____

_____

_____

8. Identify the two lasting contributions of psychoanalysis to our current understanding of depression. (page 257)

_____

_____

_____

_____

_____

9. What is "Bowlby's controversy," and what is your view of the issue? (page 257)

_____

_____

_____

_____

_____

10. What are the three types of treatment for depression? (pages 258–263)

_____

_____

_____

   a. Compare and contrast the effectiveness of these three treatment types.

_____

_____

_____

_____

_____

   b. What kinds of clients make the best candidates for each of the three types of treatment?

_____

_____

_____

_____

_____

11. Name the three classes of medication generally used to treat depression. (pages 260–263)

_____

_____

_____

   a. Identify the strengths of each class of medication.

_____

_____

_____

_____

_____

b.   Identify the drawbacks of each class of medication.

_____

_____

_____

_____

_____

c.   What education would you provide for clients taking each class of medication?

_____

_____

_____

_____

_____

12.   Identify the nursing diagnoses commonly used for clients with depression. (page 266) Be sure to differentiate between the two diagnoses related to grieving.

_____

_____

_____

_____

_____

13.   What advice would you give clients who want to use St. John's Wort (*hypericum*) to treat their depression?

_____

_____

_____

_____

_____

Self-Assessment Quiz

1. Minor Depressive Disorder is the most commonly seen DSM-IV-TR disorder. (page 251)
   - ❑ True
   - ❑ False

2. Depressions are highly treatable disorders that only infrequently persist beyond two years.
   - ❑ True
   - ❑ False

3. Major Depressive Disorder often begins in childhood. (page 250)
   - ❑ True
   - ❑ False

4. Normal grief can last as long as three years. (page 254)
   - ❑ True
   - ❑ False

5. In comparison with antidepressant medications, electroconvulsive therapy (ECT) has been shown to be the superior treatment. (pages 259–263)
   - ❑ True
   - ❑ False

6. Normal sunlight seems effective in treating Seasonal Affective Disorder. (page 260)
   - ❑ True
   - ❑ False

7. Tricyclic antidepressants can be used to treat bed-wetting, chronic pain, and migraines. (pages 260–262)
   - ❑ True
   - ❑ False

8. Prozac is usually fatal when taken in overdose. (page 262)

    ❑ True

    ❑ False

9. For a Major Depressive Episode to count toward the diagnosis of Major Depressive Disorder, it must have all the following characteristics except (page 265)

    a. Must cause the client to be sleepy and irritable

    b. Must last at least two weeks

    c. Must represent a change from previous functioning

    d. Must interfere with the client's ability to function in a social or occupational situation

10. Risk factors associated with depression include all the following except (page 266)

    a. Recent negative life stressors

    b. Concussion

    c. Significant physical disease

    d. Family history of depression

11. For cases of treatment-resistant depression, the treatment proven most effective is (page 259)

    a. allowing time to pass.

    b. electroconvulsive therapy (ECT).

    c. Prozac.

    d. MAO inhibitors.

12. All of the following classes of medications are used to treat depression except (pages 260–263)

    a. Tricyclics

    b. Amphetamines

    c. MAO inhibitors

    d. Selective serotonin reuptake inhibitors

13. Clinical problems associated with the use of tricyclics include all of the following except (page 261)

    a. Often fatal in overdose, making them problematic for clients who may be suicidal

    b. Orthostatic side effects

    c. Frequently cause insomnia and other sleep disturbances

    d. Anticholinergic side effects

14. Some recent findings of nursing research include all of the following except

    a. Exercise can be an effective antidepressant

    b. Cognitive therapy can have an antidepressant effect

    c. The ability to perform self-care has a positive effect on mood

    d. Depressed women from low socioeconomic backgrounds have a better prognosis than depressed women of affluent means

15. All of the following nursing interventions are helpful to clients with depression except (page 268)

    a. Providing overhead light 24 hours per day

    b. Cultural assessments

    c. Movement therapy

    d. Understanding the client's subjective experience of depression and pain

16. All of the following statements about St. John's Wort (*hypericum*) are true except (page 263)

    a. Some patients may be more open to taking it than standard antidepressants

    b. St. John's Wort has been shown to be as effective as drug therapy or cognitive therapy

    c. May help trigger mania in patients with unrecognized Manic-Depressive Disease

    d. St. John's Wort is an extract of a natural botanical

The Client Experiencing Mania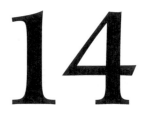

The purpose of this chapter is to gain an understanding of mania in all its forms, cycles, and manifestations. Just as depression should not be confused with the lows that sometimes accompany daily life, neither should mania be confused with the happiness, elation, and cheerfulness that all of us normally experience. When is mania pathological, and what is the nursing care associated with this complex mental illness?

Reading Assignment

Please read Chapter 14, "The Client Experiencing Mania," pages 277–301

Key Terms

Write definitions for the following terms in your own words. Compare your definitions with those given in the text on page 279.

Bipolar Disorder _____

_____

Borderline Personality ___._____

_____

Continuous Cycling _____

_____

Cyclothymic Pattern _____

_____

Hypomania _____

_____

Mania _____

_____

Manic Episode _____

_____

Rapid Cycling _____

_____

Schizoaffective Disorder _____

_____

Switch Process_____

_____

Exercises and Activities

1. In one minute, list as many adjectives as you can to describe mania.

   _____

   _____

   _____

   _____

   _____

2. Study Table 14-1, "Stages of Mania," on page 280.

   a. Cover the columns under Stage I, Stage II, and Stage III to make sure you know how mood, cognition, and behavior changes as the client moves among the stages.

   b. Identify a television character you have seen with each of the three stages of mania.

   _____

   _____

   _____

3. List the manic behaviors necessary for a diagnosis of manic episode. (page 281)

   _____

   _____

   _____

   _____

   _____

4. Differentiate among the three diagnoses manic episode, hypomania, and Bipolar Disorder. (pages 281–282)

   _____

   _____

   _____

   _____

   _____

5. Review Figure 14-1, "Clinical course of mania," on page 283.

    a. What conclusions can you draw about the frequency of episodes?

_____

_____

_____

_____

_____

    b. What conclusions can you draw about the frequency, timing, and effect of hospitalizations?

_____

_____

_____

_____

_____

6. Review Figure 14-2, "Psychologic genealogy: family with bipolar and depressive disease," on page 285.

    a. What conclusions can you draw about the nature and cause of bipolar disease?

_____

_____

_____

_____

_____

    b. According to the genealogy, in the original marriage between Elizabeth (Clayton) and Michael (Tennyson) that united the two families, the couple themselves lived lives free of mental illness. What significance has this had on their descendents?

_____

_____

_____

_____

_____

c.   What other evidence suggests that bipolar disease is genetic and biologically based?

_____

_____

_____

_____

_____

7.   What other factors can cause manic-like symptoms? (pages 286–287)

_____

_____

_____

_____

_____

8.   Complicating the diagnosis of mania is the possibility of dual diagnosis. What psychiatric conditions seem to travel in tandem with mania, making the diagnosis more problematical? (pages 287–288)

_____

_____

_____

_____

_____

9.   Describe the pharmacological treatment of mania. (pages 289–292)

_____

_____

_____

_____

_____

a. List the benefits of lithium.

_____

_____

_____

_____

_____

b. List the drawbacks of lithium.

_____

_____

_____

_____

_____

c. What teaching should nurses provide to clients taking lithium?

_____

_____

_____

_____

_____

10. If you were in charge of an inpatient setting and wanted to create a therapeutic milieu for clients with Bipolar Disorder, what features would you establish? (page 294) Think about limits, space, schedules, privileges, medication regimens, and other elements of a therapeutic milieu.

_____

_____

_____

_____

_____

Self-Assessment Quiz

1. The association between mania and depression has been observed for more than 2,000 years. (page 282)

    ❑ True

    ❑ False

2. In Bipolar Disorder, depression usually comes first, followed by the relief of mania. (page 282)

    ❑ True

    ❑ False

3. Although Bipolar Disorder is frequently seen in psychiatric settings because clients with the disease usually have repeated episodes requiring recurrent hospitalizations, the disease itself is rather rare. (page 283)

    ❑ True

    ❑ False

4. Mania almost never occurs without depression also occurring. (page 282)

    ❑ True

    ❑ False

5. Most rapid cyclers—people with at least four manic episodes in a year—are men. (page 283)

    ❑ True

    ❑ False

6. Although people in manic phases can be impulsive, they have a low risk for suicide. (page 287)

    ❑ True

    ❑ False

7. The clinical course for people with bipolar disease can vary among all the following except (page 287)

   a. Rapid cycling

   b. Mania with no depression

   c. Continuous cycling

   d. Mostly depression

8. Dual diagnoses often associated with mania include all of the following except (pages 287–288)

   a. Sociopathic Personality Disorder

   b. Substance abuse

   c. Borderline Personality Disorder

   d. Schizoaffective Disorder

9. The primary treatment for Bipolar Disorder is (page 292)

   a. psychotherapy.

   b. hospitalization and milieu therapy.

   c. channeling.

   d. medication.

10. Nursing interventions appropriate for clients with mania might include all of the following except (page 296)

    a. Milieu therapy

    b. Insight-oriented counseling and teaching about the disease when clients are between manic episodes

    c. Insight-oriented counseling and teaching about the disease when clients are experiencing manic episodes

    d. Encouraging clients to consider the benefits of lithium therapy

11.   Parse's theory of human becoming views disease as a normal part of life, something that has to be interpreted by the client, who must find individual meaning in disease as well as in health. For a nurse who approaches clinical work from this theoretical viewpoint, all of the following would be appropriate interventions except

   a.   Make no demands on the client

   b.   Help the client find and prioritize personal values

   c.   Help the client accept the health team's treatment plan

   d.   Try to understand the client's world and use that understanding to gain trust and collaboration

12.   All of the following are signs of mania except (page 282)

   a.   Increased sexual activity

   b.   Spending sprees

   c.   Carefully planned suicide attempts

   d.   Grandiose thinking

The Client Who Is Suicidal

15

The purpose of this chapter is to learn to identify clients who are at risk of suicide. Even clients who experience suicidal ideation or who make suicidal gestures to gain attention can unintentionally kill themselves in a momentary impulse or miscalculation. While suicide is associated with some disorders more than others, a wide variety of mental and physical illnesses can make people feel so awful that they might consider suicide.

Reading Assignment

Please read Chapter 15, "The Client Who Is Suicidal," pages 303–327.

Key Terms

Write definitions for the following terms in your own words. Compare your definitions with those given in the text on page 304.

Euthanasia _____

_____

Suicidal Ideation _____

_____

Suicide _____

_____

Suicide Potential _____

_____

Suicide Survivors _____

_____

Exercises and Activities

1. Who is at risk for suicide? Identify as many groups at risk discussed in this chapter as you can.

    _____

    _____

    _____

    _____

    _____

2. There is conflicting data over what percentage of people who commit suicide have a major mental illness. (page 307) After reading the chapter, what is your view?

_____

_____

_____

_____

_____

3. Nurses must be able to assess a client's potential to commit suicide. What risk factors and other conditions and circumstances can you list as concerns to assess for? (page 308)

_____

_____

_____

_____

_____

4. Peplau's theory of interpersonal relations in nursing stresses the importance of forming therapeutic relationships with clients. How can you use this nursing knowledge to reduce the likelihood of clients attempting suicide? (page 312)

_____

_____

_____

_____

_____

5. What precautions can the nurse take to protect hospitalized clients from hurting themselves? (pages 312–313)

_____

_____

_____

_____

_____

6. What precautions can the nurse take to protect clients in the community from hurting themselves? (pages 320–323)

_____

_____

_____

_____

_____

7. Describe the three levels of prevention for suicide. (pages 320–321)

_____

_____

_____

_____

_____

8. Why are listening skills effective in assessing a client's risk for suicide? (page 321)

_____

_____

_____

_____

_____

9. After reading this chapter, has your attitude changed toward the following issues? If so, in what ways? (pages 307, 317, 321–322)

   a. Gun control

_____

_____

_____

_____

_____

b. Euthanasia

_____

_____

_____

_____

_____

c. Accident rates (which may inadvertently include intentional self-harm)

_____

_____

_____

_____

_____

10. Study Vincent Van Gogh's last painting on page 312.

a. Do you agree with the author's view of elements in the painting that signify death?

_____

_____

_____

_____

_____

b. Would you be concerned if a depressed client showed you a recent painting with some of the features the author identified in Van Gogh's *Wheatfield with Crows*?

_____

_____

_____

_____

_____

    c. In what other ways do suicidal clients frequently convey their morbid thoughts of death?

_____

_____

_____

_____

_____

Self-Assessment Quiz

1. Since 1978, the incidence of teen suicide has begun to fall. (page 306)

    ❏ True

    ❏ False

2. Men over the age of 65 are the group at highest risk for suicide. (page 307)

    ❏ True

    ❏ False

3. Suicide survivors go through a similar grief process as anyone who has experienced the death of a loved one. (page 316)

    ❏ True

    ❏ False

4. Inmates serving long sentences in prisons are much more likely to commit suicide than inmates held for short periods of time in local jails. (page 316)

    ❏ True

    ❏ False

5. The trait of "openness to new experiences" has been associated with suicidal ideation. (page 307)

    ❏ True

    ❏ False

6. Explanations of suicide include all of the following except (pages 311–312)

    a. Kevorkian theory

    b. Sociological theory

    c. Psychological theory

    d. Biological theory

7. The major psychiatric diagnosis most frequently associated with suicide is (pages 309–310)

    a. Major Depressive Disorder.

    b. schizophrenia.

    c. Antisocial Personality Disorder.

    d. hypochondriasis.

8. Primary prevention of suicide includes all of the following interventions except (pages 320–321)

    a. Being aware of which groups are at greatest risk of committing suicide

    b. Limiting access to the means of suicide

    c. Using crisis intervention techniques

    d. Reducing the client's social isolation

9. A "suicide contract" is (page 322)

    a. a signed agreement between a nurse and a client in which the client promises not to commit suicide during a specific period of time.

    b. a suicide pact.

    c. a client's verbal agreement to never commit suicide without first notifying the nurse.

    d. an exclusion in a life insurance policy.

10. Tobacco use and obesity is associated with increased risk of suicide in (pages 307, 309)

    a. both men and women

    b. just men

    c. just women

    d. These factors are not significant suicide markers

The Client Who Abuses Chemical Substances

16

The purpose of this chapter is to present the psychiatric implications of substance abuse. By concentrating on the four most pervasively abused substances, though there are others, nurses can familiarize themselves with the dynamics of abuse and addiction, the effects on clients and their families, and the nursing care associated with clients who abuse substances.

Reading Assignment

Please read Chapter 16, "The Client Who Abuses Chemical Substances," pages 329–361.

Key Terms

Write definitions for the following terms in your own words. Compare definitions with those given in the text on page 331.

Addiction_____

_____

Alcoholism _____

_____

Codependence _____

_____

Craving _____

_____

Drug Dependence _____

_____

Drug Use _____

_____

Substance Abuse_____

_____

Tolerance _____

_____

Withdrawal _____

_____

Exercises and Activities

1. Terminology associated with drug abuse can be imprecise and confusing. (pages 331–332)

   a. Explain why the DSM-IV-TR uses the phrase "physiological dependence" rather than addiction.

   _____

   _____

   _____

   _____

   _____

   b. Explain the concept of tolerance.

   _____

   _____

   _____

   _____

   _____

   c. Explain the concept of withdrawal.

   _____

   _____

   _____

   _____

   _____

2. The text details efforts made by governments over the centuries to control the supply of drugs. (page 332)

   a. In your view, which if any of these measures has proven effective?

   _____

   _____

   _____

   _____

   _____

b. Besides limiting supply, governments can also act to limit demand. What efforts have governments made to limit demand?

_____

_____

_____

_____

_____

c. Have any such efforts been successful?

_____

_____

_____

_____

_____

3. In recent years, as virtually all hospitals have become "No Smoking" zones, nurses have had to manage the problem of nicotine-dependent psychiatric clients who, already stressed by their primary diseases, must abstain from smoking. (pages 335–336)

a. What specific stressors does this add to the client's burden?

_____

_____

_____

_____

_____

b. As a nurse, what can you do to help the client through this transition?

_____

_____

_____

_____

_____

4. What are the long-term adverse physical effects of chronic alcohol abuse? (pages 336–341)

_____

_____

_____

_____

5. The first task of treating clients with alcoholism is to help them withdraw from their physiological dependence on alcohol. (page 340)

   a. Describe the typical human response to alcohol withdrawal.

   _____

   _____

   _____

   _____

   _____

   b. Describe the usual medical regimen for managing the client during alcohol withdrawal.

   _____

   _____

   _____

   _____

   _____

   c. Describe measures nurses can take to help the client cope with alcohol withdrawal and the period immediately following withdrawal.

   _____

   _____

   _____

   _____

   _____

6. Describe the natural history of alcoholism. (page 340)

_____

_____

_____

_____

_____

7. Disulfiram (Antabuse) continues to be used in treating alcoholism. (page 342)

    a. Describe its mechanism.

    _____

    _____

    _____

    _____

    _____

    b. What have been the drawbacks of disulfiram?

    _____

    _____

    _____

    _____

    _____

    c. What other drugs are frequently used to treat people with alcoholism, and what are their indications?

    _____

    _____

    _____

    _____

    _____

8. Describe the Nursing "Brief Intervention" using the FRAMES Model (page 343)

_____

_____

_____

_____

_____

9. Over the years, the medical community has taken a somewhat "permissive" stance toward the use of cocaine. (pages 345–346)

   a. What are the true medical consequences of regular cocaine use?

   _____

   _____

   _____

   _____

   _____

   b. What is the DSM-IV's stance on the danger of cocaine? (page 346)

   _____

   _____

   _____

   _____

   _____

10. Review the treatment options for clients with opiate dependence. (page 348)

   a. What is the central decision clinicians must make in choosing a treatment for a person addicted to opiates?

   _____

   _____

   _____

   _____

   _____

b. Summarize the pros and cons of methadone maintenance therapy.

_____

_____

_____

_____

_____

c. What is your personal opinion of methadone maintenance therapy?

_____

_____

_____

_____

_____

11. Many public policy options are available in response to the social problem of substance abuse, ranging from long prison terms (and, in some countries, even executions) for drug users to total legalization of all chemical substances. (page 350) In your own words, state the policy you think our country should pursue.

_____

_____

_____

_____

_____

Self-Assessment Quiz

1. Drugs apparently work by activating reward centers in the brain. (page 333)

   ❑ True

   ❑ False

2. Since it ultimately causes 70 times more deaths each year than heroin and cocaine combined, it's hard not to consider nicotine an abused drug. (page 335)

   ❑ True

   ❑ False

3. Sigmund Freud was once one of the world's leading authorities on cocaine and a regular user himself. (page 344)

    ❑ True

    ❑ False

4. For those who use cocaine, withdrawal is a bigger problem than tolerance. (page 346)

    ❑ True

    ❑ False

5. Only a small percentage of people with substance abuse have another major psychiatric diagnosis. (page 350)

    ❑ True

    ❑ False

6. Among the following substances, which is not identified in the DSM-IV as a dependency psychiatric condition? (page 339)

    a. Cannabis

    b. Alcohol

    c. Caffeine

    d. Nicotine

7. Codependence refers to the relationship between (page 352)

    a. the addict and his or her dealer.

    b. two addicts or abusers.

    c. an abuser and the significant other who facilitates the substance abuse.

    d. the nurse and the substance abuser.

8. All of the following are classified as stimulants except (page 337)

    a. Nicotine

    b. Cocaine

    c. Alcohol

    d. Caffeine

9. All of the following are symptoms of untreated alcohol withdrawal except (page 338)

    a. Blackouts

    b. The shakes

    c. Hallucinations

    d. Delirium tremens

10. A recovering alcoholic should be counseled to do all of the following except (page 340)

    a. Attend AA meetings

    b. Learn how to say no to drinking alcohol at a party

    c. Deal with problems caused by drinking over the years

    d. Spend time in drinking establishments to test one's ability not to drink anymore

The Client with a Personality Disorder

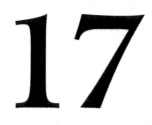

The purpose of this chapter is to better understand the concept of personality by first examining normal personality and then defects in personalities. You will learn about eleven personality disorders clustered within three types and how to be effective in providing nursing care to individuals with a personality disorder.

Reading Assignment

Please read Chapter 17, "The Client with a Personality Disorder," pages 363–397.

Key Terms

Write definitions for the following terms in your own words. Compare your definitions with those given in the text on page 365.

Antisocial Personality Disorder _____

_____

Avoidant Personality Disorder _____

_____

Borderline Personality Disorder _____

_____

Dependent Personality Disorder _____

_____

Histrionic Personality Disorder _____

_____

Narcissistic Personality Disorder _____

_____

Obsessive-Compulsive Personality Disorder _____

_____

Paranoid Personality Disorder _____

_____

Passive-Aggressive Personality Disorder _____

_____

Personality _____

_____

Personality Disorder _____

_____

Personality Traits _____

_____

Schizoid Personality Disorder _____

_____

Schizotypal Personality Disorder_____

_____

Exercises and Activities

1. Personality disorders are considered Axis II disorders in the DSM-IV, whereas most major mental illnesses are Axis I disorders. Explain the relationship between Axis II and Axis I disorders and the significance of these classifications. (page 365)

    _____

    _____

    _____

    _____

    _____

2. Almost all of us have some personality traits associated with a personality disorder. What is necessary for an individual to be diagnosed with a personality disorder? (page 365)

    _____

    _____

    _____

    _____

    _____

3. Review Table 17-1, "Personality Disorders by Descriptive Category," on page 366.

    a. What are the three clusters of personality disorders?

        _____

        _____

        _____

        _____

        _____

b. How are these clusters categorized?

_____

_____

_____

_____

_____

4. Early psychiatrists coined the term "borderline" personality because of their observations that these usually "neurotic" individuals often lived their lives on the "borderline" between neurosis and psychosis, particularly when experiencing stress. Under stress, these individuals frequently plunge into delusions, hallucinations, paranoia, and fantasies which, although they may not be persistent, are definitely psychotic. (pages 368–369)

a. List the characteristics necessary for an individual to be diagnosed with Borderline Personality Disorder.

_____

_____

_____

_____

_____

b. Identify the typical characteristics of the childhood and home life of a person diagnosed with Borderline Personality Disorder.

_____

_____

_____

_____

_____

c.   Clients with Borderline Personality Disorder can be challenging to care for. They tend to focus anger on their caregivers and blame others for their problems. They often try to "split" staff and tend to regard nurses as either allies or enemies. Since part of their illness involves a failure to form healthy relationships in their lives, it may not be surprising that they can be hard to like, and it can be hard to develop trusting therapeutic relationships with them. Considering all this, what strategies would you use to provide therapeutic nursing care to such a person?

_____

_____

_____

_____

_____

5.   Consider the personality disorders of the dramatic and emotional cluster. (pages 368–376)

a.   What is the key difference between Borderline Personality Disorder and Narcissistic Personality Disorder?

_____

_____

_____

_____

_____

b.   What are the similarities between Borderline Personality Disorder and Histrionic Personality Disorder?

_____

_____

_____

_____

c. What is the key difference between Borderline Personality Disorder and Histrionic Personality Disorder?

_____

_____

_____

_____

_____

d. People with Narcissistic Personality Disorder and people with Histrionic Personality Disorder grow up with an exaggerated sense of the importance of good looks. What life events do you think would tend to precipitate crises in these individuals? Would you expect people with the two disorders to respond any differently to these stressors?

_____

_____

_____

_____

_____

e. Clients with any of the dramatic and emotional personality disorders can place great demands on the nurse and try to use the nurse as an object in their effort to get their dysfunctional needs met. As a nurse, what strategies can you employ to minimize the demanding quality of people with these disorders?

_____

_____

_____

_____

_____

f. Although it is imperative not to stereotype individuals just because they have been diagnosed according to a set group of traits or behaviors, there is empirical evidence to show that people with Borderline Personality Disorder are more often women and people with Antisocial Personality Disorder are more often men. Do you think this trend will change as gender roles continue to evolve in society at large?

_____

_____

_____

_____

_____

6. Review the text material on the odd and eccentric cluster of personality disorders. (pages 376–379)

a. What are the essential differences between Schizoid Personality Disorder and schizophrenia?

_____

_____

_____

_____

_____

b. What is the essential difference between Schizotypal Personality Disorder and schizophrenia?

_____

_____

_____

_____

_____

c. In your own words, explain the difference between Schizoid Personality Disorder and Schizoptypal Personality Disorder.

_____

_____

_____

_____

_____

7. Characterize the difference between paranoid schizophrenia and Paranoid Personality Disorder. (page 381)

_____

_____

_____

_____

_____

8. Characterize the difference between Obsessive-Compulsive Personality Disorder and Obsessive-Compulsive Disorder, an anxiety disorder. (page 385)

_____

_____

_____

_____

_____

9. The difference between being shy and being diagnosed with Avoidant Personality Disorder is a question of degree. How would you identify the personality disorder as opposed to the personality trait? (pages 385–387)

_____

_____

_____

_____

_____

10. Have you known people who have a "passive-aggressive" style? (pages 388–390) Almost everyone has. What kinds of strategies have you developed to deal with such people?

_____

_____

_____

_____

_____

Self-Assessment Quiz

1. Personality Disorders generally develop in infancy. (page 365)

    ❏ True

    ❏ False

2. Many suicides by people with Borderline Personality Disorder are unintentional and cries for attention. (page 369)

    ❏ True

    ❏ False

3. For individuals to be diagnosed with Antisocial Personality Disorder, they must first have been diagnosable with Adolescent Conduct Disorder. (page 375)

    ❏ True

    ❏ False

4. Schizotypal Personality Disorder is probably the most common of the odd cluster of personality disorders. (page 379)

    ❏ True

    ❏ False

5. Passive-Aggressive Personality Disorder is not officially sanctioned by the DSM-IV. (page 389)

    ❏ True

    ❏ False

6. For an individual to be diagnosed with a personality disorder, all of the following must be present except

    a. Individual must experience clinically significant distress or impairment

    b. Cluster of traits must be consistent with the diagnosis

    c. Personality disorder cluster of traits must be pervasive and inflexible

    d. Personality traits must often lead to hostility and conflict

7. Strategies a nurse might use to deal with the demanding quality of clients with dramatic and emotional personality disorders include all of the following except (page 392)

    a. Setting limits on the time you devote to these clients' demands

    b. Communicating with colleagues to ensure a consistent approach toward these clients

    c. Giving these clients a little extra attention so there will be a positive feeling between you and them

    d. Responding to these clients' needs in a professional, efficient manner

8. An effective nursing response to clients with Schizoid Personality Disorder and Schizoptypal Personality Disorder might include any of the following except

    a. Designing a behavior modification program to improve social skills and increase inventory of expressive traits

    b. Accepting clients for themselves

    c. Giving clients honest feedback on how their behavior is seen by others

    d. Relating to clients in a professional, matter-of-fact manner, knowing that developing a normal relationship is inconsistent with the nature of their illness

9. In caring for a person with a Paranoid Personality Disorder, the nurse should not attempt to (page 382)

    a. respond to the client in an unemotional way.

    b. focus on the major features of the client's dysfunctional behavior.

    c. try to convince the client that paranoid feelings are unfounded.

    d. give honest feedback to the client on how the client's behavior is perceived by others.

10. Nurses should keep in mind all of the following when caring for a person with a personality disorder except (page 390)

    a. Clients with personality disorders may not be as likable as other clients with fully integrated personalities, requiring nurses to compensate for their personality deficits

    b. Clients with personality disorders respond best to clear expectations as expressed in contracts, schedules, responsibilities, and limits

    c. Clients with personality disorders benefit from honest feedback

    d. Clients with personality disorders benefit from having faithful allies on the nursing staff

The Client Experiencing a Somatoform Disorder

18

The purpose of this chapter is to understand a complex group of disorders that have the symptoms of physical diseases but have causes which lie in the psychological realm. These clients present special challenges to nursing care. They often demand that a diagnosis be made when in fact there is none to be made, and then they view their caretakers as incompetent for not curing the physical "disease." They are often unable to gain insight into their true conditions; yet, they actually feel ill—and ill treated.

Reading Assignment

Please read Chapter 18, "The Client Experiencing a Somatoform Disorder," pages 399–419.

Key Terms

Write definitions for the following terms in your own words. Compare your definitions with those given in the text on page 401.

Conversion Disorder _____

_____

Factitious Disorder _____

_____

Hypochondriasis _____

_____

Malingering_____

_____

Munchausen's Syndrome _____

_____

Munchausen's Syndrome by Proxy _____

_____

Somatization Disorder _____

_____

Somatoform Disorder _____

_____

Exercises and Activities

1. Name the four classes of disorders discussed in this chapter, briefly distinguishing one from another.

    _____

    _____

    _____

    _____

    _____

2. Somatoform disorder was once called "hysteria." (pages 402–403)

    a. What is the difference between somatoform disorder and hysteria?

        _____

        _____

        _____

        _____

        _____

    b. Why is the term *hysteria* not used in the language of psychology anymore?

        _____

        _____

        _____

        _____

        _____

3. List the four criteria for diagnosing someone with Somatization Disorder. (page 403)

    _____

    _____

    _____

    _____

    _____

4. Treatment of Somatization Disorder is notoriously difficult and frequently ineffective. Describe the nursing care that is usually associated with and sometimes effective for this disorder. (page 406)

_____

_____

_____

_____

_____

5. What are the diagnostic criteria for Hypochondriasis? (page 407)

_____

_____

_____

_____

_____

     a. How is Hypochondriasis different from the anxiety disorders?

     _____

     _____

     _____

     _____

     _____

     b. What is the key difference?

     _____

     _____

     _____

     _____

     _____

6. What are the various theories about the cause of Hypochondriasis? (page 408)

_____

_____

_____

_____

_____

a. What conclusions can you draw from the existence of these competing theories?

_____

_____

_____

_____

_____

b. In terms of your own understanding of Hypochondriasis, and as a basis for treating these clients in your nursing practice, what theory do you personally embrace?

_____

_____

_____

_____

_____

7. What can a nurse do to help a person suffering from Hypochondriasis? (pages 408–409)

_____

_____

_____

_____

_____

8. Conversion Disorder is one of the most puzzling and unimaginable of all the psychiatric disorders, and one of the hardest to treat (pages 409–411). In your view, should nurses be confrontational toward clients with Conversion Disorder? Why or why not?

_____

_____

_____

_____

_____

9. Think about your feelings toward the clients described in this chapter.

    a. Do you feel you would be angry if you were treating someone with a somatoform disorder? Why or why not?

    _____

    _____

    _____

    _____

    _____

    b. Would it make a difference in your feelings if the client had a Factitious Disorder?

    _____

    _____

    _____

    _____

    _____

    c. Sometimes it is helpful to "preadopt" an attitude toward clients with disorders like these which are treatment-resistant and a challenge to nurses. Write a statement of your preadopted attitude toward clients with somatoform disorders.

    _____

    _____

    _____

    _____

    _____

10. Clients with somatoform disorders frequently become hostile when nurses question them about their symptoms, past medical history, and stressors in their lives. (pages 413–415) Yet, these areas often produce the best assessment data.

    a. Write five assessment questions you could use to assess a client with a suspected somatoform disorder, wording them in a way that is likely to elicit the best information.

    _____

    _____

    _____

    _____

    _____

    b. List nursing diagnoses you think would be used frequently in caring for clients with somatoform disorders.

    _____

    _____

    _____

    _____

    _____

Self-Assessment Quiz

1. Once a somatoform disorder is suspected, there is no further need to vigorously explore the possibility of a physical illness. (page 406)

   ❑ True

   ❑ False

2. Successful treatment of Hypochondriasis demands that clients give up the belief that they have a serious physical disease. (page 409)

   ❑ True

   ❑ False

3. The term *Conversion Disorder* comes from the belief that a client has an underlying psychological trauma so horrendous that, rather than facing the trauma itself, the client involuntarily "converts" the trauma to a nearly equally horrific physical disability. (page 409)

   ❑ True

   ❑ False

4. Many clients with Conversion Disorder show a surprising indifference to their physical disabilities. (page 411)

    ❑ True

    ❑ False

5. Conversion Disorders often go away by themselves. (page 411)

    ❑ True

    ❑ False

6. Of the four classes of disorders discussed in this chapter, name the one that does not fit into the DSM-IV with the others.

    a. Somatization Disorder

    b. Hypochondriasis

    c. Conversion Disorder

    d. Factitious Disorder

7. All of the following are true of the incidence of Somatization Disorder except

    a. It tends to show up in families where another family member is diagnosed with Antisocial Personality Disorder

    b. The disorder is predominantly associated with women

    c. The disorder usually develops later in life

    d. The disorder is comparatively rare

8. Some of the long-used but unproven approaches to treating Conversion Disorder include all of the following except (page 411)

    a. Hypnosis

    b. Faith healing or miracle cures

    c. Forced labor

    d. Exorcism

9. When caring for a client with a Factitious Disorder, it is most helpful to keep the following in mind: (pages 412–413)

    a. Nurses should support one another when frustrated by clients with Factitious Disorder

    b. Clients with Factitious Disorder are overutilizing an already overburdened health care system

    c. Clients with Factitious Disorder take advantage of a nurse's normal caring and compassion when they fake health problems

    d. Clients with Factitious Disorder are mentally ill and in need of appropriate psychiatric care

    e. a and d

    f. a and c

10. Which of the following statements is true about Munchausen's Syndrome by Proxy? (page 412)

    a. It is a somatoform disorder, not a Factitious Disorder.

    b. Its victims are frequently the elderly.

    c. It is a form of child abuse reportable to Children's Protective Services.

    d. The father is usually the one with the mental illness.

The Client with Disorders of Self-Regulation: Sleep Disorders, Eating Disorders, Sexual Disorders

19

The purpose of this chapter is to explore the basic human functions of sleeping, eating, and sexual activity, normally associated with good mental health, and familiarize yourself with some of the more common disorders that interfere with the healthy exercise of these functions.

Reading Assignment

Please read Chapter 19, "The Client with Disorders of Self-Regulation: Sleep Disorders, Eating Disorders, Sexual Disorders," pages 421–450.

Key Terms

Write definitions for the following terms in your own words. Compare your definitions with those given in the text on pages 422–423.

Anorexia Nervosa _____

_____

Bulimia Nervosa _____

_____

Cataplexy _____

_____

Dyssomnia _____

_____

Exhibitionism _____

_____

Fetishism _____

_____

Frotteurism _____

_____

Gender Dysphoria _____

_____

Gender Identity _____

_____

Gender Identity Disorder _____

_____

Gender Role_____

_____

Hypoactive Sexual Desire Disorder_____

_____

Insomnia _____

_____

Narcolepsy _____

_____

Nightmare _____

_____

Normal Sexual Behavior _____

_____

Paraphilia _____

_____

Parasomnia _____

_____

Pedophilia _____

_____

Primary Hypersomnia _____

_____

Primary Insomnia _____

_____

Sexual Dysfunction _____

_____

Sexual Masochism _____

_____

Sexual Sadism _____

_____

Sleep Hygiene _____

_____

Sleep Latency _____

_____

Sleep Paralysis   _____

_____

Sleep Terrors   _____

_____

Sleepwalking   _____

_____

Transvestic Fetishism _____

_____

Voyeurism   _____

_____

Exercises and Activities

1. You are no doubt familiar with the biological concept of homeostasis. The lifestyle concept
    equivalent is "balance." (page 421)

    a. Explain how the disorders discussed in this chapter are related to homeostasis and
        balance.

        _____

        _____

        _____

        _____

        _____

    b. Explain how the disorders discussed in this chapter relate to health, healthiness, and
        healthy lifestyles.

        _____

        _____

        _____

        _____

        _____

2. List the factors that can interfere with normal sleep. (pages 424–429)

_____

_____

_____

_____

_____

3. How would you counsel a person with Primary Insomnia—insomnia with no apparent external cause—to improve sleep hygiene? (pages 424–426)

_____

_____

_____

_____

_____

4. What are the three major causes of daytime sleepiness, unrelated to inadequate nighttime sleep, stress, or depression? (page 427)

_____

_____

_____

_____

_____

5. How would you counsel an adolescent to promote a healthy body image? (page 433)

_____

_____

_____

_____

_____

6. Describe the negative physical and physiological consequences associated with Anorexia Nervosa. (pages 434–437)

    _____

    _____

    _____

    _____

    _____

7. Anorexia Nervosa appears to have puzzling origins. (page 436)

    a. What explanations exist for the psychological cause(s) of Anorexia Nervosa?

        _____

        _____

        _____

        _____

        _____

    b. Based on your study of the theories involved, what do you think is the cause of Anorexia Nervosa?

        _____

        _____

        _____

        _____

        _____

8. What are the three categories of sexual function disorders, and what are the differences among them? (pages 439–445)

    _____

    _____

    _____

    _____

    _____

9. What strategies would you use to make a client feel comfortable and forthcoming when you are taking a sexual history as part of an overall health assessment? (page 440)

_____

_____

_____

_____

_____

10. After reading this chapter, what do you consider to be the realm of "normal" sexual activity?

_____

_____

_____

_____

_____

Self-Assessment Quiz

1. As an age group, the elderly—those over age 65—have the fewest sleep disturbances. (page 426)

   ❑ True

   ❑ False

2. Narcolepsy is more common than sleepwalking. (pages 428–429)

   ❑ True

   ❑ False

3. Bulimia Nervosa and Anorexia Nervosa can both be present in the same individual. (page 433)

   ❑ True

   ❑ False

4. Nurses rarely actually witness bingeing and purging behavior (page 433)

   ❑ True

   ❑ False

5. Whether an issue of sexuality is a "disorder" or not is partially dependent on how problematic it is for the individual or couple involved. (page 440)

    ❑ True

    ❑ False

6. Which of the following statements about normal sleep is true? (page 424)

    a. Although sleep deprivation causes people to feel unwell, there are no known serious adverse physiological consequences of sleep deprivation in an otherwise healthy person.

    b. There may be five stages of normal sleep, but the average person rarely goes through all five in a single night.

    c. It is a myth that sleep patterns change in old age.

    d. Scientists are on the verge of discovering all the secrets of sleep.

7. All of the following are primarily sleep disorders of children and adolescents, rather than adults, except (pages 424–429)

    a. Narcolepsy

    b. Night terrors

    c. Sleepwalking

    d. Nightmares

    e. a and b

    f. a and c

    g. a and d

8. All of the following are disorders of sexual functioning except (pages 439–445)

    a. Sadism

    b. Hypoactive Sexual Desire Disorder

    c. Premature ejaculation

    d. Erectile disorder

9. All of the following are widely recognized paraphilias except (page 442)

    a. Voyeurism

    b. Pedophilia

    c. Fraterphilia

    d. Exhibitionism

10. None of the following are recognized in the DSM-IV as disorders except

    a. Gender Identity Disorder

    b. Heterosexuality

    c. Hyperactive Sexual Desire Disorder

    d. Homosexuality

The Physically Ill Client Experiencing Emotional Distress

20

The purpose of this chapter is to reinforce the point that virtually every person facing a serious physical disease experiences emotional stress, which can lead to symptoms of mental illness. Understanding the connections between the body and the mind is key to developing appropriate nursing care. The skills of psychiatric nursing are indispensable to the effective practice of nursing in virtually all settings.

Reading Assignment

Please read Chapter 20, "The Physically Ill Client Experiencing Emotional Distress," pages 453–475.

Key Terms

Write definitions for the following terms in your own words. Compare your definitions with those given in the text on page 454.

Liaison Psychiatry/Liaison Psychiatric Nursing _____

_____

Mind Modulation _____

_____

Exercises and Activities

1. State your beliefs about the body-mind connection. (page 453)

   _____

   _____

   _____

   _____

   _____

2. How does the DSM-IV handle the connection between serious physical illnesses and major mental illnesses? (page 456)

   _____

   _____

   _____

   _____

   _____

3. Read the Reflective Thinking box about reactions to very ill clients on page 458. If you found that your personal feelings interfered with your ability to effectively care for a particular client, what measures would you pursue to deal with the situation?

_____

_____

_____

_____

_____

4. Read the story of Dr. Lear's heart attack on pages 461–462.

   a. What efforts did Dr. Lear make to maintain control over his situation?

   _____

   _____

   _____

   _____

   _____

   b. Were these efforts to maintain control therapeutic, destructive, or both?

   _____

   _____

   _____

   _____

   _____

   c. What interventions by others did Dr. Lear find comforting?

   _____

   _____

   _____

   _____

   _____

d. Did these interventions interfere with his need to maintain control over his situation?

_____

_____

_____

_____

_____

5. What interventions can a nurse perform to treat a family member who has the nursing diagnosis of caregiver role strain?

_____

_____

_____

_____

_____

6. Write a job description for a liaison psychiatric nurse. (pages 471, 472)

_____

_____

_____

_____

_____

7. Study Table 20-1, "Summary of Nursing Process . . . ," on page 473.

a. Do you agree with the correlations suggested between the nursing process and Erickson's theory?

_____

_____

_____

_____

_____

b. Consulting the list of NANDA nursing diagnoses in Appendix D on pages 817–818, make a list of nursing diagnoses that would be commonly used for a client having difficulty adapting to a severe physical illness.

_____

_____

_____

_____

_____

8. The fact that most heart attacks occur on Mondays is often cited as evidence for a strong body-mind connection. Can you think of other evidence for this phenomenon?

_____

_____

_____

_____

_____

9. Look up stress in your medical surgical or pathophysiology textbook. What evidence does it cite to support an explanation of stress (General Adaptation Syndrome) based on the new science of psychoneuroimmunology? Record the highlights here.

_____

_____

_____

_____

_____

10. Nurses, it is said, are at the forefront in understanding and making use of the body-mind connection. Why do you think this is a significant domain for nurses?

_____

_____

_____

_____

_____

Self-Assessment Quiz

1. This chapter focuses on case studies because each person's illness and response to illness is unique.

   ❑ True

   ❑ False

2. Experience has shown that humor, touch, companionship, natural, and other nonmedical types of interventions have no effect on the outcome of physical illnesses.

   ❑ True

   ❑ False

3. Many of the negative medical outcomes experienced by a client with a disease come about as a result of the client's response to a disease rather than as a result of the disease itself.

   ❑ True

   ❑ False

4. All nursing theories call upon nurses to view the client holistically.

   ❑ True

   ❑ False

5. Although nurses frequently refer to the body-mind connection, physicians reject such a connection due to the lack of physiological evidence.

   ❑ True

   ❑ False

6. All of the following are measures nurses can use to establish trust except (page 473)

   a. Set aside time to spend with clients

   b. Keep appointments with clients

   c. Read each client's chart

   d. Keep promises made to clients

7. Mind modulation refers to (page 473)

   a. the mechanism with which the body transforms thoughts, emotions, attitudes, and images into neurohormonal messenger molecules.

   b. the use of sound waves to affect brain waves.

   c. a nursing theory that helps clients cope with stress.

   d. psychosurgery.

8. Mr. Davies may have died as a result of his mental illness not being treated after his second heart attack. His DSM-IV diagnosis should have been

   a. mood disorder due to a general medical condition.

   b. Major Depressive Disorder as an Axis I diagnosis without any Axis III diagnosis.

   c. Major Depressive Disorder as an Axis I diagnosis with an Axis III diagnosis of diseases of the circulatory system (myocardial infarction).

   d. hopelessness.

9. Which of the following measures is *not* an example of offering a client "unconditional acceptance"?

   a. Helping clients identify personal strengths

   b. Planning to spend unstructured time with clients

   c. Pointing out that better health habits might have prevented the current illness

   d. Providing interventions that enhance comfort

10. Emily Dickinson wrote, "Hope is a thing with feathers." In his book *Without Feathers*, Woody Allen noted that hopelessness can be fatal. Nurses can foster the healing power of hope in a client experiencing hopelessness by all of the following except

    a. Forming a caring relationship with the client

    b. Reassuring the client that everything will turn out all right

    c. Helping the client regain control over health-related decision making

    d. Helping the client make lifestyle adaptations that will help facilitate recovery or adapt to the client's changing health state

Forgotten Populations: The Homeless and the Incarcerated

21

The purpose of this chapter is to focus on two demographic groups with high rates of mental illness, the homeless and the incarcerated. While prisoners usually have access to excellent health care services, homeless people generally do not.

Reading Assignment

Please read Chapter 21, "Forgotten Populations: The Homeless and the Incarcerated," pages 477–491.

Key Terms

Write definitions for the following terms in your own words. Compare your definitions with those given in the text on page 478.

Deinstitutionalization _____

_____

Homelessness _____

_____

Incarcerated_____

_____

NIMBY Syndrome _____

_____

Exercises and Activities

1. Read the chapter opening box, "Walking Down the Street," on page 477.

    a. Write down your personal responses to the homeless and to the incarcerated.

    _____

    _____

    _____

    _____

    _____

b. Regardless of your personal views, which to some extent reflect your values, is there anything that would hold you back from providing members of these groups the same quality of nursing care you would provide to anyone else?

_____

_____

_____

_____

_____

2. Name four factors that have contributed to the increase in homelessness since 1975. (page 480)

_____

_____

_____

_____

_____

3. If you are old enough to have this perspective, do you personally agree that homelessness has increased considerably since 1975, compared to years earlier? One of the culprits is the deinstitutionalization of the chronically mentally ill. Deinstitutionalization had been going on since the 1950s, however; what made the problem of homelessness so much worse after 1975?

_____

_____

_____

_____

_____

4. Name the major health problems of homeless people. (pages 481–484)

_____

_____

_____

_____

5. Consulting the list of NANDA nursing diagnoses in Appendix D on pages 817–818, list those nursing diagnoses that would be likely to have the most frequent application to the homeless.

    _____

    _____

    _____

    _____

    _____

6. What are the major health problems faced by people in prison? (page 487)

    _____

    _____

    _____

    _____

    _____

7. The United States may have the highest percentage of its population in prisons and jails of any country on earth, with more than 1 million incarcerated adults expected by the year 2000. What factors contribute to this situation? (page 487)

    _____

    _____

    _____

    _____

    _____

8. What conditions present the greatest risk of suicide among the incarcerated? (pages 487–488)

    _____

    _____

    _____

    _____

    _____

9. In what ways can nurses be effective advocates for the homeless and the incarcerated? (page 489)

_____

_____

_____

_____

10. Identify the homeless shelter closest to where you live. Volunteer at the shelter to learn more about the extent of the homeless problem in your community and the specific factors and problems affecting your local homeless population.

Self-Assessment Quiz

1. It is important for the nurse to assess each homeless person as an individual with unique problems and strengths.

   ❏ True

   ❏ False

2. It is possible for the nurse to assess the needs of groups within the community of homeless people and design treatment programs that would benefit all members of the group. (page 486)

   ❏ True

   ❏ False

3. The lack of a permanent residence is not a major factor in providing social services to homeless people.

   ❏ True

   ❏ False

4. Until recently, the United States has done a better job of providing social services to "worthy" homeless people than to "unworthy" homeless people.

   ❏ True

   ❏ False

5. Schizophrenia is more prevalent among the homeless than substance abuse and alcoholism. (page 481)

   ❑ True

   ❑ False

6. The lack of safety, cleanliness, and privacy affect the homeless and the incarcerated alike.

   ❑ True

   ❑ False

7. A year at Harvard is cheaper than a year in prison. (page 486)

   ❑ True

   ❑ False

8. The ANA Standards of Nursing Practice for working in correctional facilities mandate all the following except (page 488)

   a. Facilitating inmates' contact with the outside world

   b. Ensuring inmates' human rights

   c. Ensuring equal access to health services for all inmates

   d. Ensuring equal quality health care for all inmates

9. The Clubhouse Model has been successful because (page 483)

   a. Mentally ill people prefer to socialize among themselves

   b. It substitutes for a happier childhood

   c. It reduces isolation among homeless and mentally ill people

   d. It meets the needs of the homeless and mentally ill while eliminating the need to find gainful employment

10. All of the following are grounds for involuntary commitment to a locked mental health facility except

   a. Severe psychotic thought processes

   b. Demonstrated risk of harm to self

   c. Demonstrated risk of harm to others

   d. Demonstrated total inability to care for basic self needs

The Child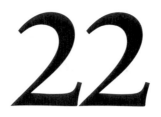

The purpose of this chapter is to review the major psychiatric disorders of childhood which, like the medical diseases of childhood, differ significantly in type and character from adult disorders. Inasmuch as children cannot choose their living circumstances in the way adults can, they present special challenges to the mental health community, and their care cannot always be separated from the mental health care of their caregivers.

Reading Assignment

Please read Chapter 22, "The Child," pages 493–519.

Key Terms

Write definitions for the following terms in your own words. Compare your definitions with those given in the text on page 494.

Asperger's Syndrome _____

_____

Autism _____

_____

Conduct Disorder _____

_____

Dysthymia _____

_____

Oppositional Defiant Disorder _____

_____

Reactive Depression _____

_____

Separation Anxiety _____

_____

Social Phobia _____

_____

Exercises and Activities

1. Most adults have positive feelings toward children who are loveable and well behaved. In mental health settings, however, you will encounter children who are less approachable and may exhibit unlikable behavior. State in your own words your usual response to children like this.

   _____

   _____

   _____

   _____

   _____

2. What are the DSM-IV-TR diagnostic criteria for Attention-Deficit Hyperactivity Disorder (ADHD)? Think it terms of number of symptoms, variety of settings, age of onset, and functional impairment. (page 497)

   _____

   _____

   _____

   _____

   _____

3. Treatment of ADHD is termed "Multi-Modal." Describe a complete treatment program for a child with ADHD. (page 498)

   _____

   _____

   _____

   _____

   _____

4. Think about what you learned about the major mood disorders in chapter 13, Major Depressive Disorder, Dysthymic Disorder, and Bipolar Disorder.

    a. What differences are seen, if any, when these disorders are manifested in children?

    _____

    _____

    _____

    _____

    _____

    b. What differences in efficacy are seen, if any, in the treatments available for adults and children—particularly young children—for major mood disorders?

    _____

    _____

    _____

    _____

    _____

5. What factors would you include in assessing the seriousness of a child's suicidal ideation or behavior? (page 500)

    _____

    _____

    _____

    _____

    _____

6. Separation anxiety is quite normal for an infant or toddler. What characteristics make it pathological? (page 502)

    _____

    _____

    _____

    _____

    _____

7. For the following anxiety disorders, identify the ones found almost always only in childhood with a "C," and those found both in children and adults with an "A." Indicate the forms of effective treatment.

	Drug Therapy	**Other Tx**
Attention Deficit/Hyperactivity Disorder	_____	_____
Generalized Anxiety Disorder	_____	_____
Separation Anxiety	_____	_____
Social Phobia	_____	_____
Obsessive-Compulsive Disorder	_____	_____

8. Differentiate Asperger's syndrome from Autism. What treatments, if any, seem efficacious? (page 000)

    _____

    _____

    _____

    _____

    _____

9. A continuum of severity, from less disruptive to more disruptive, exists among Oppositional Defiant Disorder (ODD), Conduct Disorder, and Antisocial Personality Disorder. (page 507)

    a. How would you differentiate among these disorders?

        _____

        _____

        _____

        _____

        _____

b. What risk factors may contribute to these developmental disorders?

_____

_____

_____

_____

_____

c. What treatment options seem viable for each of these Disruptive Disorders?

_____

_____

_____

_____

_____

10. Read the Case Study about "Jean" on page 513. What do you think her DSM-IV diagnosis would be?

_____

_____

_____

_____

_____

Self-Assessment Quiz

1. Children experience mental illness in much the same way as adults do. (page 495)

    ❑ True

    ❑ False

2. Stimulants used to treat Attention-Deficit Hyperactivity Disorder work by increasing the availability of dopamine. (page 498)

    ❑ True

    ❑ False

3. Children can be tested for the presence of Attention Deficit Hyperactivity Disorder. (page 497)

    ❑ True

    ❑ False

4. Optimal treatment for ADHD includes both pharmacologic and psychosocial modalities. (page 498)

    ❑ True

    ❑ False

5. Reactive Depression is the kind that doesn't require treatment. (page 500)

    ❑ True

    ❑ False

6. The manic phase of Bipolar Disorder in children is differentiated from ADHD by (page 501)

    a. Hyperactive behavior is episodic or cyclical

    b. It responds to Ritalin

    c. Bipolar Disorder does not occur until late adolescence

    d. Children with Bipolar Disorder do not allow their behavior to get them in trouble as children with ADHD do

7. All of the following are normal expressions of Separation Anxiety except (pages 502–503)

    a. A 3-year-old has to stay overnight at the home of a family friend due to an emergency

    b. A 6-year-old has experienced several traumatic events

    c. A pre-teen is exceptionally shy

    d. A 9-year-old won't go to camp or sleep at a friend's house

8. Which of the following criteria is appropriate for considering a diagnosis of Conduct Disorder? (page 508)

    a. Isolated acts of misbehavior

    b. Antisocial behavior beyond what would be expected in normal growth and development

    c. Socioeconomic status

    d. School performance

9. The most effective treatment of Conduct Disorder is (page 508)

    a. caregiver management training in behavior shaping programs.

    b. haldol or lithium therapy.

    c. individual therapy.

    d. incarceration.

10. All of the following are risk factors for childhood emotional disorders except (page 509)

    a. Physical disability of child

    b. Poverty

    c. Caregiver psychopathology

    d. Divorce

11. Play therapy is used for all the following therapeutic purposes except (page 511)

    a. Caregiver training

    b. Exploring relationships

    c. As a substitute for verbal interaction

    d. Attempting new solutions to problems

The Adolescent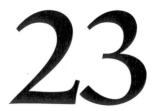

The purpose of this chapter is to understand the most turbulent time of human development, the transition from childhood to adulthood known as adolescence. You should become familiar with the mental health disorders associated with this period and be able to differentiate the mental health problems of adolescence from the normal turbulence of adolescence.

Reading Assignment

Please read Chapter 23, "The Adolescent," pages 521–547.

Key Terms

Write definitions for the following terms in your own words. Compare your definitions with those given in the text on page 523.

Foreclosure _____

_____

Gender Identity _____

_____

Gender Role_____

_____

Identity Achievement _____

_____

Identity Diffusion _____

_____

Identity Formation _____

_____

Identity Status_____

_____

Moratorium_____

_____

Presence _____

_____

Self-awareness _____

_____

Self-efficacy _____

_____

Social Competence _____

_____

Suicidal Ideation _____

_____

Exercises and Activities

1. Read the chapter opening box on page 521.

    a. What problems did you experience in adolescence?

    _____

    _____

    _____

    _____

    _____

    b. Do you think it is harder to go through adolescence today than it was during your adolescent years? In what ways?

    _____

    _____

    _____

    _____

    _____

    c. How did your current sense of personal identity develop during your adolescence? Has it changed since? In what ways?

    _____

    _____

    _____

    _____

    _____

2. Adolescence is characterized by cognitive changes and decision making that may be characterized by lack of impulse control, risk taking, and lack of regard for long-term consequences. List problems that often result from this feature of adolescence.

    _____

    _____

    _____

    _____

    _____

3. Identify the three stages of adolescence; include descriptors. (page 526)

    _____

    _____

    _____

    _____

    _____

4. Review Table 23-1, "Four Statuses of Adolescent Identity," on page 527.

    a. Which status best reflects your own adolescence?

        _____

        _____

        _____

        _____

        _____

    b. Can you visualize adolescents you have known who fit into the other statuses?

        _____

        _____

        _____

        _____

        _____

5. Middle adolescents often conform to their peers in their search for what's "normal." How would you counsel such an adolescent in terms of explaining what's normal for the age group?

_____

_____

_____

_____

_____

6. Read "When Rabbit Howls" on page 531.

   a. What is your reaction to Truddi?

   _____

   _____

   _____

   _____

   _____

   b. Do you think she experienced suicidal ideation?

   _____

   _____

   _____

   _____

   _____

7. Summarize the risk factors associated with adolescent suicide. (page 533)

_____

_____

_____

_____

_____

8. List some strategies for talking with an adolescent therapeutically about sex. (page 535)

_____

_____

_____

_____

_____

9. How would you teach an adolescent about how to prevent AIDS and other STDs?

_____

_____

_____

_____

_____

10. Test your knowledge of adolescent culture by making a list of current expressions, musicians, and popular culture icons currently favored by adolescents.

_____

_____

_____

_____

_____

11. Explain in your own words what humanistic nursing is. (page 536)

_____

_____

_____

_____

_____

12. What measures could you use to establish rapport with an adolescent whose racial or ethnic identity is different from your own?

_____

_____

_____

_____

_____

Self-Assessment Quiz

1. The central task of adolescence is identity formation. (page 526)

    ❑ True

    ❑ False

2. Suicide is the second leading cause of death among adolescents. (page 530)

    ❑ True

    ❑ False

3. Not every suicidal expression or gesture should be taken seriously. (page 530)

    ❑ True

    ❑ False

4. In dealing with adolescents, it's a good idea to familiarize yourself with the language, music, and popular culture currently in vogue.

    ❑ True

    ❑ False

5. Over 50% of adolescents are unsure of their sexual orientation. (page 534)

    ❑ True

    ❑ False

6. In Newman's framework, the focus of nursing is not on the treatment of the disease but on helping clients understand the meaning of their pattern of health and how it fits into the scheme of the universe. (page 538)

   ❑ True

   ❑ False

7. Social competence is a concept characterized by (page 540)

   a. choosing friends wisely.

   b. having good manners.

   c. decoding, interpreting, and responding to social cues.

   d. being able to move easily among social classes.

8. All of the following psychiatric disorders can originate in adolescence except

   a. Schizophrenia

   b. Autism

   c. Conduct Disorder

   d. Anorexia Nervosa

9. Warning signs of potential adolescent suicide include (page 533)

   a. increased risk taking, interest in shaving, and upcoming important dates.

   b. previous suicidal gestures, giving away possessions, and getting an after-school job.

   c. expression of wish to die, stated feelings of sadness or despair, and sudden deterioration of behavior or appearance and hygiene.

   d. alienating behavior, preoccupation with death or dying, and mild disappointment.

10. Which of the following assessment findings would make a nurse feel concerned about the mental health of an adolescent client? (page 539)

    a. Inability to concentrate on tasks at hand; numbness or lack of affect; inability to maintain eye contact

    b. Inability to tolerate young children; constant wearing of earphones; using vulgar or provocative language

    c. Constant fidgeting; anger and hostility; admiration for rock stars

    d. Inability to maintain eye contact; rolls eyes when mother speaks; wants to drive the family car

11. Statistically, adolescents are at the greatest risk for developing mental health problems if they are

   a. from single-caregiver families in which the caregiver has a history of mental problems.

   b. from middle-class homes.

   c. smoking cigarettes before age 12.

   d. never going to learn to drive.

12. Studies show that the main factor that protects adolescents best from dangerous and risky behavior is

   a. good genes.

   b. connectedness with parents and school.

   c. desire for attention.

   d. character traits such as will power.

The Elderly

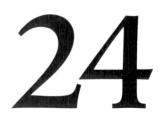

The purpose of this chapter is to gain an appreciation for the unique mental health needs and problems experienced by the elderly. It also includes a discussion of the needs of those who are charged with caring for the elderly.

Reading Assignment

Please read Chapter 24, "The Elderly," pages 549–583.

Key Terms

Write definitions for the following terms in your own words. Compare your definitions with those given in the text on page 551.

Aphasia _____

_____

Catastrophic Reaction _____

_____

Cognition _____

_____

Confabulation _____

_____

Confusion _____

_____

Delirium _____

_____

Dementia _____

_____

Mutuality _____

_____

Exercises and Activities

1. Many older people who become victims of dementia actually recognize the early signs of failing memory and coming dysfunction. (page 566)

   a. If you recognized these early symptoms in yourself, what treatment would you seek?

   _____

   _____

   _____

   _____

   _____

   b. What precautions would you take, or what alterations would you make in your daily functioning?

   _____

   _____

   _____

   _____

   _____

   c. What legal, financial, and family decisions would you make?

   _____

   _____

   _____

   _____

   _____

2. Identify the four types of cognitive disorders in the elderly and define them. (page 553)

   _____

   _____

   _____

   _____

   _____

3. Differentiate among delirium, confusion, and acute confusional states. What is the terminology appropriate for health care professionals? (page 554–556)

_____

_____

_____

_____

_____

4. Define "dignity" in your own words.

_____

_____

_____

_____

_____

    a. What measures could you implement to help preserve the dignity of a client who was being placed in a nursing home against the client's wishes?

_____

_____

_____

_____

_____

    b. What measures could you implement to help preserve the dignity of a client who needed assistance with dressing, eating, toileting, or walking?

_____

_____

_____

_____

_____

c. What measures could you implement to help preserve the dignity of a client who had been placed in restraints?

_____

_____

_____

_____

_____

5. Review the Geriatric Depression Scale on page 562. What score is indicative of depression?

_____

_____

_____

_____

_____

6. Name the four subtypes of depression and differentiate them from one another. (pages 559–561)

_____

_____

_____

_____

_____

7. Read the poem "Survived by His Wife" on page 561. Explain why the author compares the possessions of the dead husband to "frames of stolen paintings left behind."

_____

_____

_____

_____

_____

8. Define "self-transcendence" and its relationship to risk for suicide. (page 563)

_____

_____

_____

_____

_____

9. Research is making progress in helping to explain the origins and pathophysiology of Alzheimer's Disease. (pages 567–568)

    a. Differentiate between Early-onset and Late-onset Alzheimer's Disease. What seems to be the cause of the Early-onset variety?

_____

_____

_____

_____

_____

    b. Two defining findings associated with Alzheimer's Disease are beta-amyloid plaques and neurofibrillary tangles. Why do these processes seem to be so debilitating? What seems to cause them?

_____

_____

_____

_____

_____

    c. What treatments may contribute to slowing down the course of Alzheimer's Disease?

_____

_____

_____

_____

_____

d. What treatments may delay the onset or prevent Alzheimer's Disease?

_____

_____

_____

_____

_____

e. What seems to be the effect of brain infarction on Alzheimer's Disease?

_____

_____

_____

_____

_____

10. Write a script of a conversation with an older person with dementia, identifying when the client is confabulating. (page 570)

_____

_____

_____

_____

_____

Self-Assessment Quiz

1. Alzheimer's disease is often cited as the number one mental health problem affecting the aging population. (pages 566–567)

   ❏ True

   ❏ False

2. Major features of a client's personality usually are not totally submerged and are often exaggerated by dementia.

   ❏ True

   ❏ False

3. The "old-old," people over the age of 85, are the slowest growing age group in the population. (page 551)

    ❑   True

    ❑   False

4. Depression is the most common mental health problem of old age. (page 558)

    ❑   True

    ❑   False

5. Grief is a mood disorder commonly seen in the elderly. (page 560)

    ❑   True

    ❑   False

6. Alzheimer's Disease can only be diagnosed through autopsy.

    ❑   True

    ❑   False

7. All of the following can cause dementia except (page 567)

    a. Schizophrenia

    b. Syphilis

    c. Parkinson's disease

    d. Head injury

8. All of the following are typical behaviors associated with dementia except (pages 571–573)

    a. Paranoia

    b. Hypochondria

    c. Aggression

    d. Wandering

9. The best strategy for understanding a client with aphasia would be to (page 572)

    a. ask the client to repeat himself until you understand.

    b. repeat something that sounds to you like what the client said.

    c. ask "yes" and "no" questions to clarify what the client wants.

    d. smile and reassure the client.

10. Nurses can help caregivers of clients with dementia in all the following ways except (pages 574–577)

    a. Explaining the diagnosis honestly and frankly

    b. Encouraging the making of legal and financial decisions as soon as possible, with the participation of the client if possible

    c. Encouraging the client and caregiver to participate in insight-oriented therapy

    d. Making the caregiver aware of community resources

11. Nurses can help caregivers to accept their decision to place a loved one in a nursing home by all of the following except (pages 579–580)

    a. Encouraging the caregiver to take a cruise or "do something for yourself for a change"

    b. Helping the caregiver see any humor there may be in the situation

    c. Pointing out that the client will adapt to the nursing home over time

    d. Reminding the caregiver that the nursing home may be in a position to provide better care for the client than the client could have continued to get at home.

Survivors of Violence or Abuse

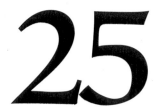

The purpose of this chapter is to focus on the care of victims of violence, our most serious social problem. Understanding the dynamics of relationships that spark violence helps to promote safety and health care. Victims of violence and abuse often require special health care. This chapter helps the psychiatric nurse to provide care needed by this large group of victims.

Reading Assignment

Please read Chapter 25, "Survivors of Violence or Abuse," pages 585–629.

Key Terms

Write definitions for the following terms in your own words. Compare your definitions with those given in the text on page 587.

Acquaintance (or Date) Rape _____

_____

Aggravated Criminal Sexual Assault _____

_____

Child Abuse_____

_____

Child Molestation _____

_____

Child Pornography _____

_____

Criminal Sexual Assault _____

_____

Domestic Violence _____

_____

Financial Abuse _____

_____

Forcible Rape _____

_____

Gang Rape _____

_____

Incest _____

_____

Mental Injury _____

_____

Negligent Treatment _____

_____

Passive Physical Abuse (or Negligence) _____

_____

Physical Abuse _____

_____

Physical Injury _____

_____

Psychological Abuse _____

_____

Rape _____

_____

Sexual Abuse (Child) _____

_____

Sexual Abuse (Elder) _____

_____

Sexual Battery _____

_____

Sexual Exploitation _____

_____

Sexually Explicit Conduct _____

_____

Spousal Rape _____

_____

Statutory Rape _____

_____

Stranger Rape _____

_____

Violation of Rights _____

_____

Exercises and Activities

1. Review Table 25-1, "Common Myths about Rape," on pages 599–600. List the myths that you previously believed.

    _____

    _____

    _____

    _____

    _____

2. Nurses are usually required to report domestic violence to the authorities when they become aware of it. When fulfilling this legal obligation, nurses should take what precautions to protect the survivor in the coming crisis? (page 614)

    _____

    _____

    _____

    _____

    _____

3. Some victims of domestic violence feel trapped and stay with their tormenter; others find the wherewithal to leave the abusive relationship. (pages 603–609)

    a. List the circumstances which can be helpful for an abused partner to seriously consider leaving the abuser.

    _____

    _____

    _____

    _____

b. List the reasons many abused partners cannot bring themselves to leave their abusers.

_____

_____

_____

_____

_____

c. How would you counsel a battered partner who doesn't feel able to leave the batterer?

_____

_____

_____

_____

_____

4. What information should be included in a child abuse report? (page 591)

_____

_____

_____

_____

_____

5. Review the characteristics and symptoms of child abuse on pages 594 and 595. Design an assessment tool you could use to help identify children at risk for abuse.

_____

_____

_____

_____

_____

6. Study Figure 25-1, "The Power and Control Wheel," on page 604.

    a. Why are power and control at the center of the wheel?

    _____

    _____

    _____

    _____

    _____

    b. Explain ways in which an abuser can wield power and control.

    _____

    _____

    _____

    _____

    _____

7. Describe the three phases in the common pattern of domestic violence. (pages 605–607)

    _____

    _____

    _____

    _____

    _____

8. Explain how Orem's self-care deficit theory can be applied to survivors of abuse and neglect. (pages 613–614)

    _____

    _____

    _____

    _____

    _____

9. Compare and contrast the criteria for the NANDA diagnosis of post-trauma syndrome and the DSM-IV-TR diagnosis for Post-Traumatic Stress Disorder. (pages 618–619)

_____

_____

_____

_____

_____

10. Were you ever in a situation when you felt a loss of control and another person had complete power and control over your personal safety and well-being? Try to reconstruct the kinds of feelings any client might feel in such a situation.

_____

_____

_____

_____

_____

Self-Assessment Quiz

1. Both the survivor and the perpetrator of domestic abuse tend to have low self-esteem. (page 605)

   ❑ True

   ❑ False

2. Women who stay in violent relationships are more likely to be murdered than women who leave their violent spouse. (page 608)

   ❑ True

   ❑ False

3. Adolescents are less at risk for abuse than younger, more defenseless children. (page 595)

   ❑ True

   ❑ False

4. Rape is a medical diagnosis. (page 597)

   ❑ True

   ❑ False

5. Passive physical abuse is the same thing as negligence. (page 609)

   ❑ True

   ❑ False

6. The three phases of the common pattern of domestic violence include all of the following except the (pages 605–607)

   a. Tension-building phase

   b. Irrational thoughts stage

   c. Acute battering incident

   d. Loving reconciliation

7. The 1992 Joint Commission on the Accreditation of Healthcare Organizations (JCAHO) required written protocols for emergency and ambulatory care units that cover all of the following except (page 614)

   a. Making referrals to forensic nurses

   b. Obtaining informed consent from abused clients

   c. Handling possible evidence

   d. Making referrals to resources in the community

8. Guidelines for effective nursing care of abused clients include all of the following except (page 615)

   a. Providing privacy

   b. Being nonjudgmental

   c. Expressing outrage about the client's ordeal

   d. Using active and empathic listening skills

9. The following federal agencies and initiatives play an active role in the prevention of violence:

   a. The FBI and the federal Bureau of Prisons

   b. The Bureau of the Census and the Veterans Administration

   c. The Administration on Aging and the National Institutes of Health

   d. Healthy People 2010 and the U.S. Public Health Services

10. Objectives for preventing violence and abuse which Congress incorporated into Healthy People 2010 include all of the following except (page 625)

    a. Reduction of weapons carried by adolescents on school property

    b. Reduction of the number of deaths of children resulting from abuse

    c. Raising the level of civility in public discourse, including radio and television

    d. Lowering the number of rapes

Pharmacology in Psychiatric Care

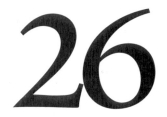

The purpose of this chapter is to familiarize you with psychopharmacology and the pharmacological treatment of clients with psychiatric disorders. Drug therapy has become the dominant mode of treatment for many forms of mental illness, and it is an area of intensive research and rapid development. It is essential to understand the pharmacological action and nursing considerations associated with each major drug class and many widely used individual drugs. It is also important to know how to find drug information when you need it, and when you need to teach your clients about the medications they are taking.

Reading Assignment

Please read Chapter 26, "Pharmacology in Psychiatric Care," pages 633–667.

Key Terms

Write definitions for the following terms in your own words. Compare your definitions with those given in the text on page 635.

Akathisia _____

_____

Antipsychotic Drugs _____

_____

Blood-Brain Barrier _____

_____

Dystonia _____

_____

Half-Life _____

_____

Neuroleptic Malignant Syndrome _____

_____

Oculogyric Crisis _____

_____

Serotonergic Syndrome _____

_____

Tardive Dyskinesia _____

_____

Therapeutic Window _____

_____

Exercises and Activities

1. Name the seven chemical classes of antipsychotic drugs. (page 639)

   _____

   _____

   _____

   _____

   _____

   a. Which of these are the "classical drugs"?

   _____

   _____

   _____

   _____

   _____

   b. Of the newer drugs, which group has shown the most promise?

   _____

   _____

   _____

   _____

   _____

2. Review the drug actions of antipsychotics on page 642.

   a. What are the two actions associated with antipsychotic drugs?

   _____

   _____

   _____

   _____

   _____

b. How are antipsychotics similar to and different from narcotics and sedatives?

_____

_____

_____

_____

_____

c. Characterize the benefits and drawbacks of risperidone.

_____

_____

_____

_____

_____

d. If haloperidol is less expensive than the atypical neuroleptics, why did the author suggest that treatment with atypical neuroleptics might be less expensive overall?

_____

_____

_____

_____

_____

3. What are the main adverse effects resulting from use of antipsychotics? (page 643)

_____

_____

_____

_____

_____

4. Name the four classes of drugs used to treat mood disorders. (page 645)

    _____

    _____

    _____

    _____

    _____

5. When a client is given a tricyclic antidepressant, how long will it take for the client to feel relief from depression? (page 646)

    _____

    _____

    _____

    _____

    _____

    a. What symptoms may improve before the depression itself improves?

        _____

        _____

        _____

        _____

        _____

    b. What side effects should the nurse be alert to?

        _____

        _____

        _____

        _____

        _____

6. What considerations should the clinician take into account when deciding what kind of antidepressant should be prescribed for a client with a clinical depression? (pages 645–648)

_____

_____

_____

_____

_____

7. How would you counsel a client who is experiencing unpleasant side effects from antidepressants and wants to discontinue using them?

_____

_____

_____

_____

_____

8. Teaching clients about medications is an important nursing function.

   a. What teaching would you provide to a client who has been prescribed an MAO inhibitor?

   _____

   _____

   _____

   _____

   _____

   b. What teaching would you provide to a client who has been prescribed lithium?

   _____

   _____

   _____

   _____

   _____

9. Why are so many new antidepressants coming onto the market? What characterizes these new antidepressants?

_____

_____

_____

_____

_____

10. Briefly state the advantages of the following medications:

a. Buspirone (BuSpar)

_____

_____

_____

_____

_____

b. Zolpidem (Ambien)

_____

_____

_____

_____

_____

c. Propranolol (Inderal)

_____

_____

_____

_____

_____

11. Why do people respond differently to the same drugs, and why do drugs cause different side effects—or no side effects at all—in different people?

_____

_____

_____

_____

Self-Assessment Quiz

1. Neuroleptics are the same thing as antipsychotics. (page 639)

   ❑ True

   ❑ False

2. The negative symptoms of schizophrenia do not respond to classical antipsychotics, although they may respond to atypical antipsychotics like Clozaril. (page 638)

   ❑ True

   ❑ False

3. When drugs are assigned a pregnancy risk category of "X," indicating that animal and human studies have demonstrated fetal abnormalities or adverse effects, the clinician may decide that the potential benefits of giving the drug outweigh the potential risks. (page 638)

   ❑ True

   ❑ False

4. Prozac is an example of an antidepressant that acts upon serotonin-related pathways. (page 648)

   ❑ True

   ❑ False

5. All medications used in the treatment of anxiety and insomnia are benzodiazepines. (page 657)

   ❑ True

   ❑ False

6. Olanzapine is a new atypical antipsychotic that may not produce the potentially fatal side effect of agranulocytosis, the major drawback of Clozapine. (page 639)

   ❑ True

   ❑ False

7. Disadvantages of current antipsychotic drugs include all the following except

   a. They control symptoms, but they don't cure diseases

   b. Many people with the most severe symptoms are not helped by the currently available drugs

   c. The currently available drugs can cause devastating side effects

   d. Many currently available antipsychotics are also used to treat other health problems

8. It is believed that many psychotropic drugs are effective because (pages 637–638)

   a. their molecules are too large to pass the blood-brain barrier.

   b. they bond to proteins.

   c. they bind to brain receptors for dopamine.

   d. they cannot modify neurotransmitters.

9. The safest antidepressant to prescribe to a pregnant or lactating woman is

   a. No antidepressant should ever be prescribed to a pregnant or lactating woman

   b. Cyclic antidepressants

   c. An SSRI

   d. MAO inhibitors

10. The drug-receptor hypothesis is the (page 664)

   a. theory that some people are more receptive to drug effects than others.

   b. theory that drugs bind at the molecular level to receptor sites in the human body.

   c. fact that drugs can be given in a variety of routes, such as orally, by injection, or intravenously.

   d. belief that drugs will be abused unless regulated by the FDA.

11. Stimulants can be effective and prudent medications for all of the following conditions except (page 663)

    a. Depression

    b. Narcolepsy

    c. Fatigue

    d. Adult Attention-Deficit Disorder

12. Identify the following drugs as either antipsychotics (P), antidepressants (D), or antianxiety (A) medications.

    _____ Risperdal

    _____ Elavil

    _____ Loxitane

    _____ Klonopin

    _____ Librium

    _____ Ambien

    _____ Mellaril

    _____ Desyrel

    _____ Prozac

    _____ Thorazine

    _____ BuSpar

    _____ Haldol

    _____ Ativan

    _____ Olanzapine

Individual Psychotherapy

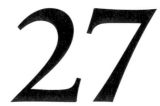

The purpose of this chapter is to help you understand the effectiveness of individual psychotherapy as a treatment for psychiatric disorders. In this chapter, you will learn which disorders are effectively treated with this modality, as well as the techniques associated with individual psychotherapy. The various modes and methods of individual therapy are discussed, and the unique role of nurses in providing individual therapy is presented.

Reading Assignment

Please read Chapter 27, "Individual Psychotherapy," pages 669–681.

Key Terms

Write definitions for the following terms in your own words. Compare your definitions with those given in the text on page 671.

Catharsis _____

_____

Clarification _____

_____

Client-Centered Therapy _____

_____

Cognitive-Behavioral Therapy _____

_____

Confrontation _____

_____

Experience-Oriented Therapy _____

_____

Insight-Oriented Therapy _____

_____

Interpersonal Therapy _____

_____

Interpretation _____

_____

Manipulation _____

_____

Psychoanalysis _____

_____

Psychodynamic Therapy _____

_____

Psychotherapy _____

_____

Repression _____

_____

Suggestion _____

_____

Task-Oriented Therapy _____

_____

Exercises and Activities

1. The difference between psychotherapy and counseling can be vague. What is the difference as you understand it? (pages 671–672)

    _____

    _____

    _____

    _____

    _____

2. Which health professionals are licensed to perform psychotherapy? (pages 671–672)

    _____

    _____

    _____

    _____

    _____

    a. What qualifications does a therapist have to have?

        _____

        _____

        _____

        _____

        _____

b. What kinds of psychotherapy and/or counseling is a nurse entitled to provide, and what qualifications must the nurse have? Be sure to consider your state's Nurse Practice Act.

_____

_____

_____

_____

_____

3. Think about Salvatore Dali's painting on page 672.

a. Why do you think Dali called it *The Persistence of Memory*?

_____

_____

_____

_____

_____

b. What is it about psychoanalysis that led the authors to offer this painting as a pictorial analogy to psychotherapy?

_____

_____

_____

_____

_____

4. List the pros and cons of intensive psychoanalysis, as you see them. (pages 672–673)

a. Pros

_____

_____

_____

_____

_____

b. Cons

_____

_____

_____

_____

_____

5. Compare and contrast Freudian psychoanalytic therapy with Rogerian client-centered therapy. (pages 672–676)

_____

_____

_____

_____

_____

6. Identify nursing theories that are consistent with the role of the nurse as individual therapist and provide a brief rationale. (pages 678–679)

_____

_____

_____

_____

_____

7. In a collaborative psychiatric setting, who are the other mental health professionals on the team? (page 679)

_____

_____

_____

_____

_____

a. What are their roles and responsibilities?

_____

_____

_____

_____

_____

b. Which of these roles and responsibilities could be assumed by a nurse in advanced practice?

_____

_____

_____

_____

_____

c. What are the unique roles and responsibilities of the nurse on the team?

_____

_____

_____

_____

_____

8. As suggested on page 677, you can find many forms of therapy in any Internet search, stroll through a bookstore, or a late night spent channel surfing on cable TV, and many are practiced or advocated by people outside the mainstream of the established mental health profession.

a. How would you counsel a client who inquires about the usefulness of a new, nontraditional form of therapy?

_____

_____

_____

_____

_____

b. What laws, if any, would you like to see passed to regulate the practice of individual therapy?

_____

_____

_____

_____

_____

c. Inasmuch as government regulations tend to limit choices for consumers, how could you justify government regulation of the practice of individual therapy?

_____

_____

_____

_____

_____

9. Cite evidence supporting the efficacy of cognitive behavioral therapy.

_____

_____

_____

_____

10. Study Table 27-1, "Techniques Used in Psychoanalysis," on page 673.

a. Try to give another example of each technique, based on experiences you have had with clients and practitioners.

_____

_____

_____

_____

_____

b. Do you think any of these techniques could and should be used by nurses engaged in short-term individual therapy with clients?

_____

_____

_____

_____

_____

Self-Assessment Quiz

1. Long-term intensive psychoanalysis is an example of an insight-oriented therapy. (page 673)

    ❏   True

    ❏   False

2. Cognitive-behavioral therapy is an example of an insight-oriented therapy. (page 674)

    ❏   True

    ❏   False

3. Cognitive-behavioral therapy would be of little use in treating a person with depression. (page 675)

    ❏   True

    ❏   False

4. Even in this era of emphasis on the biological basis of mental illness and the use of medications to treat it, individual therapy has consistently proven to be an effective treatment for many types of mental illness. (page 677)

    ❏   True

    ❏   False

5. The nursing process, although crucial to other areas of nursing practice, is not used in the practice of psychotherapy. (page 678)

    ❏   True

    ❏   False

6. Besides intensive psychotherapy, people today can choose from a variety of approaches to therapy, organized according to all of the following categories except (pages 672–676)

   a. Experience-oriented therapies

   b. Denial-oriented therapies

   c. Insight-oriented therapies

   d. Task-oriented therapies

7. Characteristics of cognitive-behavioral therapy include all of the following except (page 674)

   a. Understanding the origins of current problems

   b. Short-term duration

   c. Oriented toward self-help

   d. Practical results oriented

8. All of the following are true statements about interpersonal therapy except (page 674)

   a. Client mental health problems arise in the course of human relationships rather than in individual psychodevelopment

   b. The therapy is based on the ideas of Sullivan, not Freud

   c. Nurses can substitute for poor relationships elsewhere in the client's life

   d. Nurses can model positive relationships using Peplau's theory

9. All of the following are techniques of psychoanalysis except (page 673)

   a. Coercion

   b. Confrontation

   c. Manipulation

   d. Suggestion

10. Cognitive-behavioral therapy can be used effectively with all the following psychiatric disorders except (page 675)

    a. Substance abuse

    b. Eating disorder

    c. Psychotic thought patterns

    d. Sexual dysfunction

Family Therapy

28

The purpose of this chapter is to explore the role of families in psychiatric mental health nursing. Individuals with mental health problems can both affect and be affected by their families. Nurses need to understand family development and dynamics, and to develop skills associated with assessing and intervening with families to promote health, prevent illness, and treat problems.

Reading Assignment

Please read Chapter 28, "Family Therapy," pages 683–709.

Key Terms

Write definitions for the following terms in your own words. Compare your definitions with those given in the text on page 685.

Circular Communication _____

_____

Differentiation_____

_____

Ecomap _____

_____

Emotional Cutoff _____

_____

Family _____

_____

Family Attachment Diagram _____

_____

Family Projection Process _____

_____

Genogram _____

_____

Interventive Questions _____

_____

Multigenerational Transmission Process _____

_____

Nuclear Family Emotional System _____

_____

Power _____

_____

Relativistic Thinking _____

_____

Sibling Position _____

_____

Societal Regression _____

_____

Triangulation _____

_____

Exercises and Activities

1. The definition of family is very broad. (page 685)

   a. For the purposes of providing effective nursing care, why must this be so?

   _____

   _____

   _____

   _____

   _____

   b. In cases where family membership is ambiguous, how can the nurse determine who are family members?

   _____

   _____

   _____

   _____

c. Do you hold any value judgments about what a family is that you think could interfere with your ability to provide care to a family group? What decisions can you make right now that would enable you to provide professional nursing care if a client's family values clashed with your own?

_____

_____

_____

_____

_____

2. Review Table 28-1, "Four Approaches to Family Nursing in Psychiatric Mental Health Care," on page 687. Cover the middle column and define each approach's use in psychiatric nursing in your own words. Check yourself with the information given in the table.

3. Using your family or a family close to you as an example, answer the following questions about family development (pages 688–689):

a. What stage of family development is your family in?

_____

_____

_____

_____

_____

b. What tasks must your family master before moving on to the next stage?

_____

_____

_____

_____

_____

c. In what ways, if any, would Duvall's Family Development Theory be inadequate to sufficiently account for current developmental issues in your family? (page 688)

_____

_____

_____

_____

_____

4. Study Table 28-3, "Level of Differentiation and Family Patterns," on page 691.

a. Explain the general differences among families in terms of low, moderate, and high level of differentiation.

_____

_____

_____

_____

_____

b. What application does the concept of differentiation have to caring for families?

_____

_____

_____

_____

_____

5. Using the figures presented on page 695, draw a genogram of your family, carrying it out to three generations.

6. Using your family genogram, make a family attachment diagram, using yourself as the focal point. (page 695)

7. Explain the relationship between family assessment and family intervention. (pages 694–700)

_____

_____

_____

_____

_____

8. Draw an ecomap with your family in the middle. (pages 695–696)

a.   What surprised you about your family's ecomap?

_____

_____

_____

_____

_____

b.   What changes would you like to make, if any, in the strength of connections between various elements in your family's ecomap?

_____

_____

_____

_____

_____

9.   Think about the trifocal model in terms of your family. (page 696)

a.   What are the wellness patterns in your family?

_____

_____

_____

_____

_____

b.   What areas of prevention do you think your family would benefit from?

_____

_____

_____

_____

_____

c. What family problems can you identify in your family?

_____

_____

_____

_____

_____

10. List NANDA nursing diagnoses which, although originally developed to be applied to individuals, might also be used with family units. (pages 696–698)

_____

_____

_____

_____

_____

Self-Assessment Quiz

1. Relativistic thinking is a negative characteristic in family processes. (page 690)

    ❑ True

    ❑ False

2. Structural family theory seeks to explain how families adapt to or find a new equilibrium to accommodate dysfunctional or unhealthy family behavior. (page 692)

    ❑ True

    ❑ False

3. In the trifocal model, the same nursing diagnosis can be used whether the family is in a state of wellness, could benefit from prevention, or is in need of problem resolution. (page 696)

    ❑ True

    ❑ False

4. Circular communication refers to unpredictable patterns of communication that interfere with family processes. (page 694)

    ❑ True

    ❑ False

5. It is rare for a family problem to be caused by family problems that existed in a generation before the immediately previous generation.

    ❑ True

    ❑ False

6. A modern definition of family would exclude the following individual(s) from membership in the family: (page 686)

    a. People not related by blood

    b. People not living together

    c. Disinherited children

    d. People who the family members agree are not part of the family

7. Families with a low level of differentiation are characterized by (page 690)

    a. acting like 2-year-olds.

    b. acting impulsively, emotionally, and selfishly.

    c. lack of ability to function is all aspects of life.

    d. intense but short-term relationships.

8. The following are among Bowen's concepts of familial and emotional interaction patterns except (page 688)

    a. Strangulation

    b. Triangulation

    c. Emotional cutoff

    d. Differentiation

9. Nurses can positively affect families in all of the following ways except (page 688)

    a. Nurses can help identify family strengths

    b. Nurses can identify and point out patterns and rules within families that may be unhealthy but unseen by the family itself

    c. Nurses can become a surrogate member of the family

    d. Nurses can identify the source of individual problems within the context of family problems

10. All of the following family perspectives are useful to the nurse except (pages 686–687)

    a. Family as a component of society

    b. Family as a political group

    c. Family as context

    d. Family as client

Group Therapy

The purpose of this chapter is to explain how groups can accomplish therapeutic purposes and to show nurses the techniques and approaches to group work that can help facilitate positive outcomes.

Reading Assignment

Please read Chapter 29, "Group Therapy," pages 711–725.

Key Terms

Write definitions for the following terms in your own words. Compare your definitions with those given in the text on page 712.

Closed Group _____

_____

Group _____

_____

Group Content _____

_____

Group Dynamics _____

_____

Group Leader/Facilitator _____

_____

Group Process _____

_____

Open Group _____

_____

Self-Help Group _____

_____

Supportive Group _____

_____

Therapy Group _____

_____

Exercises and Activities

1. Name as many different kinds of client groups as you can think of. (page 713)

_____

_____

_____

_____

_____

2. Review Table 29-1, "Three Phases of Group Work," on page 713. Compare these stages with Peplau's interpersonal relations in nursing stages, page 717.

_____

_____

_____

_____

_____

3. In your own words, state the "roles" that help facilitate the group process. (page 716)

_____

_____

_____

_____

_____

4. An effective technique that nurses can use to facilitate groups is to comment on the group process. Compose a facilitating statement to respond to the following situations (page 716):

   a. The group has gotten off track.

_____

_____

   b. The group has fallen silent.

_____

_____

c. Two members of the group are arguing.

_____

_____

d. One member of the group is dominating.

_____

_____

e. One member of the group is not participating verbally but is making many nonverbal and body language gestures.

_____

_____

f. One member of the group is not participating verbally or nonverbally.

_____

_____

g. All the group members seem to be hostile toward or unsupportive of one group member.

_____

_____

h. One group members is hostile toward or argumentative with all other group members.

_____

_____

5.   You may be familiar with television shows that depict group therapy. Even though the shows are intended to be funny or dramatic, the group therapy is intended to mimic real therapy approaches. To the best of your ability, identify the group therapy approaches used in the following shows, explaining the rationale for your answer.

a.   *Frasier* (radio show, "I'm listening . . . ")

_____

_____

_____

_____

_____

b.   *The Bob Newhart Show* (psychologist conducts group therapy in his office)

_____

_____

_____

_____

_____

c.   *Dear John* (a divorced man in a support group for divorcees)

_____

_____

_____

_____

_____

6.   A self-help group is formed for people seeking support and solutions from peers facing similar problems. List client problems you have seen in your clinical experience that you think might benefit from the formation of a self-help group. (page 721)

_____

_____

_____

_____

_____

7. Give examples of "socialization" groups you or your parents or significant others may have arranged for you when you were growing up whose purpose it was to help you approach some developmental task. (page 720)

_____

_____

_____

_____

_____

8. What kind(s) of group would an Outward Bound or wilderness survival experience be? (pages 720–721)

_____

_____

_____

_____

_____

9. What is the purpose of silence in a group?

_____

_____

_____

_____

_____

10. Explain the difference between group process and group dynamics. (page 715)

_____

_____

_____

_____

_____

Self-Assessment Quiz

1. Very often two group leaders can facilitate a group better than one group leader. (page 716)
   - ❑ True
   - ❑ False

2. In a therapy group, the nurse should not usually follow the nursing process. (page 717)
   - ❑ True
   - ❑ False

3. The nurse is licensed and trained to lead many kinds of groups. (page 716)
   - ❑ True
   - ❑ False

4. Reminiscence groups work well with any adult age group. (page 720)
   - ❑ True
   - ❑ False

5. According to the ANA, nurses who function as group therapists should have a master's degree. (page 716)
   - ❑ True
   - ❑ False

6. All of the following are valid approaches to therapy groups except (pages 717–718)
   a. Existential groups
   b. Interpersonal groups
   c. Psychodrama
   d. Confessional approach

7. All of the following are self-help groups except (page 721)
   a. Overeaters Anonymous
   b. Motivational seminars
   c. Fund-raisers
   d. Grief groups

8. The reasons that psychoanalytic therapy can work well in a group include all of the following except (page 717)

   a. Clients may be unwilling to disclose embarrassing personal information in a group setting

   b. Clients may feel empowered to disclose embarrassing personal information if they see that someone else was able to do so and be supported

   c. Clients may receive more varied and helpful feedback to their disclosures

   d. Clients may come to understand that they are not alone in their feelings

9. Psychodrama is an effective group modality for many clients for all these reasons except: (pages 719–720)

   a. It is impossible for the client to hide from past disturbing events by erecting a barrier to years of feelings, denials, and repression

   b. Reliving past uncomfortable events is accomplished in a safe, supportive setting

   c. It offers clients an opportunity to change or alter past traumatic experiences

   d. It offers clients an opportunity to achieve closure to past traumatic experiences

10. The group leader who reaches the termination phase of a group should do all of the following except (pages 714–715)

    a. Planning for the group's termination, perhaps by organizing a ceremony or small party

    b. Recognizing that feelings of change, sadness, and anxiety may accompany the termination of a group

    c. Suggesting or planning a group reunion at a future date so that it does not really feel as if the group is terminating

    d. Asking members to state the ways they may have benefited from being part of the group

Community Mental Health Nursing

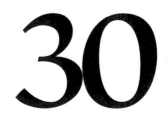

The purpose of this chapter is to help you understand how the concept of community health nursing can be applied to psychiatric/mental health nursing. Community psychiatric/mental health nursing is of particular importance following the massive deinstitutionalization in the 1970s of people severely ill with mental illness, shifting the need for psychiatric nursing resources from hospitals to the community.

Reading Assignment

Please read Chapter 30, "Community Mental Health Nursing," pages 727–741.

Key Terms

Write definitions for the following terms in your own words. Compare your definitions with those given in the text on page 728.

Aggregate _____

_____

Capitation _____

_____

Case Management _____

_____

Community Health Nursing_____

_____

Community Mental Health _____

_____

Community Support System (CSS) _____

_____

Deinstitutionalization _____

_____

Home Health Nursing _____

_____

Managed Care_____

_____

Population _____

_____

Primary Prevention _____

_____

Program for Assertive Community Treatment (PACT)_____

_____

Prospective Payment System _____

_____

Public Health Nursing _____

_____

Secondary Prevention _____

_____

Tertiary Prevention_____

_____

Exercises and Activities

1. What resources exist in your community to care for people with mental illnesses? (page 731)

    _____

    _____

    _____

    _____

    _____

2. Add important legislation that led to the creation of mental health resources in the community to your time line. (page 730)

3. What kind of nursing support is needed by individuals with schizophrenia who function adequately when taking their medication? (pages 730–731)

    _____

    _____

    _____

    _____

    _____

4. Define case management. (page 731)

    _____

    _____

    _____

    _____

    _____

    a. List the six areas of responsibility for case managers.

        _____

        _____

        _____

        _____

        _____

    b. Provide examples of these six areas of responsibility.

        _____

        _____

        _____

        _____

        _____

5. Compare and contrast a community support system (CSS) with a Program for Assertive Community Treatment (PACT). (pages 731–733)

    _____

    _____

    _____

    _____

    _____

6. What kinds of community mental health services are essential to serve this unique population? (page 733)

_____

_____

_____

_____

_____

7. What are the rights of people with mental illnesses? (page 734)

_____

_____

_____

_____

_____

8. Patient's rights is a topic of ongoing public debate.

    a. What are the latest developments?

    _____

    _____

    _____

    _____

    _____

    b. Do any of these developments pertain to the rights of people with mental illness?

    _____

    _____

    _____

    _____

    _____

9. List the stressors experienced by family members caring for relatives with mental illnesses. (page 735)

_____

_____

_____

_____

_____

   a. How should community mental health agencies address the needs of caregivers?

     _____

     _____

     _____

     _____

     _____

   b. What can nurses do to ease the burden of caregivers?

     _____

     _____

     _____

     _____

     _____

10. What responsibilities, roles, and tasks are associated with the position of psychiatric home care provider?

_____

_____

_____

_____

_____

Self-Assessment Quiz

1. Inadequate community resources following massive deinstitutionalization in the late 1960s and 1970s resulted in the creation of community support systems (CSSs). (page 736)

   ❑ True

   ❑ False

2. The "politically correct" term for the chronically mentally ill, once *long-term mentally ill,* has now evolved to *seriously mentally ill.* (page 734)

   ❑ True

   ❑ False

3. The case management model is most effective for people with a dual diagnosis or in need of multiple services. (page 735)

   ❑ True

   ❑ False

4. Capitation limits the provider's, not the insurer's, financial responsibility for the consumption of mental health services. (page 736)

   ❑ True

   ❑ False

5. Case management is a type of managed care. (page 736)

   ❑ True

   ❑ False

6. The founder of modern public health or community health nursing is

   a. Florence Nightingale.

   b. Hildegard Peplau.

   c. Lillian Wald.

   d. Margaret Sanger.

7. Many social forces work against successful care of the mentally ill population in the community. (pages 733–735) These forces include all of the following except

    a. Unqualified or unwilling caregivers in the clients' families

    b. Discrimination against people with mental illness

    c. Health insurance company practices

    d. Mental health advocacy groups

8. The mission of the National Alliance for the Mentally Ill (NAMI) includes all of the following except (page 733)

    a. Establish civil rights for people with mental illness

    b. Promote deinstitutionalization

    c. Fight against the stigmatization of the mentally ill

    d. Lobby governments for more effective legislation for the treatment of people with psychiatric disorders

9. All of the following statements about the public health model are true except (page 736)

    a. The community, not the individual, is the focus of treatment

    b. The model does not apply to populations of people who are already severely mentally ill

    c. The emphasis of the model is on prevention

    d. The concept of prevention can apply to people who are already severely mentally ill

10. In the twenty-first century, psychiatric nurses working in the community will face all of the following challenges except (page 738)

    a. Care will be increasingly collaborative

    b. Nurses working with the mentally ill in the community will be paid better than social workers, psychologists, and nurses working in hospitals

    c. Nurses will focus more on rehabilitative services

    d. Nurses will work more often for managed-care firms

Complementary and Somatic Therapies

31

The purpose of this chapter is to familiarize the nurse with the somatic therapies long used in psychiatric care and the generally newer complementary therapies used mainly by nurses to add to the diversity of medical and psychiatric therapies. These interventions and treatments augment conventional psychiatric practice and nursing and broaden the scope of psychiatric nursing. All of the complementary therapies are classified as nursing interventions by NIC and have been shown to be effective in treating specific psychiatric disorders and symptoms.

Reading Assignment

Please read Chapter 31, "Complementary and Somatic Therapies," pages 743–757.

Key Terms

Write definitions for the following terms in your own words. Compare your definitions with those given in the text on page 745.

Anger Control Assistance _____

_____

Animal-Assisted Therapy _____

_____

Complementary Modalities _____

_____

Electroconvulsive Therapy (ECT) _____

_____

Energy-Based Modalities _____

_____

Guided Imagery _____

_____

Healing Touch_____

_____

Hypnosis _____

_____

Light Therapy (Phototherapy) _____

_____

Massage _____

_____

Music Therapy _____

_____

Relaxation _____

_____

Seclusion _____

_____

Somatic Therapies _____

_____

Therapeutic Imagery _____

_____

Therapeutic Massage _____

_____

Therapeutic Touch (TT) _____

_____

Exercises and Activities

1. When you feel overwhelmed with stress, how do you treat yourself? What relaxes you?
    (pages 745–747)

    _____

    _____

    _____

    _____

    _____

2. What characteristics of Frederick Varley's painting Dhârâna, on page 746, suggest
    relaxation?

    _____

    _____

    _____

    _____

3. Read the material on guided imagery on pages 747–748.

    a. What are the differences between guided imagery and relaxation therapy?

    _____

    _____

    _____

    _____

    _____

    b. What is the pleasant "place" in your mind which you would visit if you were practicing guided imagery on yourself?

    _____

    _____

    _____

    _____

    _____

    c. What techniques can be used to enhance the effectiveness of guided imagery?

    _____

    _____

    _____

    _____

    _____

    d. What are some characteristics of people who can image responsively?

    _____

    _____

    _____

    _____

    _____

4. What are your state's licensing, educational, and supervisory requirements to practice hypnosis or hypnotherapy?

_____

_____

_____

_____

_____

5. What is the difference between massage and therapeutic massage? (page 749)

_____

_____

_____

_____

_____

a. What training have you received in massage as a nursing student?

_____

_____

_____

_____

_____

b. What conditions can be treated effectively with therapeutic massage?

_____

_____

_____

_____

6. The authors state, "Simple touch—reaching out to physically contact another—is a therapy too often neglected in busy nursing practice." Do you agree? Why or why not? (page 749)

_____

_____

_____

_____

_____

7. Have you ever used music therapy to treat a sleep disturbance you have experienced? If so, what aspects of your self-treatment did you find effective? (pages 751–752)

_____

_____

_____

_____

_____

8. What signals are there that a client is at risk for becoming violent? (page 753)

_____

_____

_____

_____

_____

9. Review the material on physical restraints on page 753.

   a. What requirement must be satisfied before physical restraints can be used?

   _____

   _____

   _____

   _____

   _____

b. What techniques are associated with the therapeutic or safe and professional use of restraints on clients?

_____

_____

_____

_____

_____

c. What message should be directed toward a client who is being restrained?

_____

_____

_____

_____

_____

d. What conditions and practices must be observed while a client is in restraints?

_____

_____

_____

_____

_____

10. When is electroconvulsive therapy (ECT) indicated? (pages 754–755)

_____

_____

_____

_____

_____

a. What is your personal opinion of ECT?

_____

_____

_____

_____

_____

b. What are the risks of ECT?

_____

_____

_____

_____

_____

c. Considering how painful mental illness can be, has your opinion of ECT changed since you began this course but before you read this chapter? If so, in what ways?

_____

_____

_____

_____

_____

Self-Assessment Quiz

1. When practiced skillfully by trained nurses on clients for whom it is not contraindicated, relaxation therapy and guided imagery can cause no harm. (page 748)

   ❑ True

   ❑ False

2. Hypnotherapy is the use of hypnosis to resolve psychic trauma and distress. (page 749)

   ❑ True

   ❑ False

3. Martha Rogers developed therapeutic touch. (page 750)

    ❑ True

    ❑ False

4. The best music to achieve a relaxation response in music therapy has a strong rhythm with beats that are slower than the heart rate. (page 752)

    ❑ True

    ❑ False

5. Electroconvulsive therapy (ECT) has been proven effective in reducing violent behavior in people with schizophrenia. (pages 754–755)

    ❑ True

    ❑ False

6. The physiological changes that take place during relaxation therapy include all of the following except (page 746)

    a. One becomes aware that one has been tense or stressed

    b. The parasympathetic nervous system gains dominance over the sympathetic nervous system

    c. Blood pressure, heart rate, and respiratory rate are decreased

    d. Alpha waves in the brain are increased

7. Guided imagery should never be used with people who are (page 748)

    a. going through labor and childbirth.

    b. experiencing psychotic thought processes.

    c. experiencing pain.

    d. depressed.

8. Music therapy is used for (page 751)

    a. entertainment.

    b. diversion.

    c. measurable relaxation response.

    d. reducing anxiety in the operating room.

9. All of the following are true of electroconvulsive therapy (ECT) except (pages 754–755)

   a. Nobody knows why it works

   b. It seems most effective in clients with depression and bipolar illness

   c. It should be used to punish incorrigible clients because it works by means of a guilt mechanism

   d. A controlled seizure seems to produce the therapeutic effect

10. Post-ECT nursing care includes all of the following except (page 755)

    a. Monitoring brain activity with electroencephalograms

    b. Orienting client to time, place, and person

    c. Monitoring vital signs

    d. Monitoring behavior, including confusion, until short-term memory returns to normal

Self-Care Modalities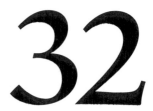

The purpose of this chapter is to help you develop knowledge and techniques designed to reduce the stress of caring for clients with psychiatric disorders. Not surprisingly, many of the techniques and modalities that nurses use to reduce stress in clients can be used in self-care to prevent burnout, protect one's own health, and open up new horizons and opportunities in the practice of nursing.

Reading Assignment

Please read Chapter 32, "Self-Care Modalities," pages 762–777.

Key Terms

Write definitions for the following terms in your own words. Compare your definitions with those given in the text on page 762.

Burnout _____

_____

Circadian Rhythm _____

_____

Parasympathetic System Response _____

_____

Sympathetic System Response _____

_____

Victim Consciousness _____

_____

Exercises and Activities

1. Have you ever watched a movie and left the theater feeling as if you had the power and charisma of the film's heroine or hero? Have you ever felt energized in the presence of a vivacious, charismatic, enthusiastic, elated, or cheerful person? (pages 764–765) Do you believe it is possible for you to create such positive feelings in a client through the personal magnetic power of your own presence? Can you give any examples of these phenomena?

_____

_____

_____

_____

2. The authors reference several books written by nurses that document their attraction to nursing and the odysseys they have taken in pursuing their careers. (pages 763–765) Have you read any other books by either nurses or clients that document their stories, aspirations, or struggles to achieve peacefulness, contentment, and reward in their lives?

_____

_____

_____

_____

_____

3. Make a list of factors you think can contribute to nurse burnout.

_____

_____

_____

_____

_____

4. What does the acronym "HALT" stand for? Give an example of how you might use this technique as an internal self-assessment.

_____

_____

_____

_____

_____

5. Name the six modalities nurses can use to refresh their physical, emotional, mental, and spiritual health and enhance their stamina and nursing performance. (pages 766–774)

_____

_____

_____

_____

_____

6. How do the forces associated with burnout affect your energy field? (pages 770–771)

    _____

    _____

    _____

    _____

    _____

    a. How can you restore health to the energy field that surrounds you?

        _____

        _____

        _____

        _____

        _____

    b. How can your clients benefit from a healthy vibrant energy field radiating from your physical presence?

        _____

        _____

        _____

        _____

        _____

7. Activities like centering may seem "far out" or unscientific, and many nurses are skeptical about trying this technique. However, agree to suspend your judgement and practice centering, described on page 771, for a full day the next time you are in a clinical setting. Then, record the results of your experiment here.

    _____

    _____

    _____

    _____

    _____

8. Form a support group with some peers where you can practice the kinds of support interventions you all agree are most helpful. Ban griping and designate someone to be the "energy monitor." (page 774) What interventions are most effective?

_____

_____

9. With a group of your peers, listen to and discuss a motivational audiotape like Napoleon Hill's "Think and Grow Rich." (page 773) Which strategies do you find to be most motivational?

_____

_____

10. Interview your peers to try to learn at least three new self-care techniques or insights today. (page 774) List the three techniques you think are best here.

_____

_____

_____

Self-Assessment Quiz

1. Since the thirteenth century, nurses have sacrificed themselves to the care of their clients; unfortunately, this is a necessary condition of the nursing profession. (page 765)

   ❑ True

   ❑ False

2. Optimal attentiveness lasts only 90 to 120 minutes in most people. (page 765)

   ❑ True

   ❑ False

3. Although meditation may seem "far out" or exotic to many who grew up in the Western world, it has long been an accepted and effective practice in the religions and cultures of the Eastern world. (page 768)

   ❑ True

   ❑ False

4. Martha Rogers expanded the concept of energy fields (like magnetism) in physics to explain the interconnectedness of all beings. (pages 770–771)

   ❑ True

   ❑ False

5. Humor can be especially helpful when dealing with psychotic clients, clients with a different cultural background, clients who speak little English, or clients who have just received bad news. (page 773)

   ❑ True

   ❑ False

6. The personal benefits of imagery include all of the following except (pages 766–768)

   a. The benefits can be had within one minute, in any location

   b. It can allow nurses to reconnect to their inner resources

   c. It isolates nurses from their colleagues and clients

   d. It can restore a sense of health and balance

7. Techniques that facilitate meditation and deep relaxation include all of the following except (pages 768–769)

   a. Any repetitive task as it can be conducive to meditation if the individual accepts the task as a joy in itself

   b. Breathing exercises

   c. Visualizing the peaceful inner workings of your healthy body

   d. Reviewing past injustices you have suffered

8. A positive outcome of meditative self-care or self-hypnosis might be that (page 769)

   a. you can get by on less sleep if you meditate.

   b. you don't need to seek medical attention for a health problem if you try to heal yourself with your own mind.

   c. you can let your subconscious do your thinking for you.

   d. you might open your mind to new solutions to old problems.

9. All of the following are essential to centering except (pages 770–771)

    a. Standing with squared shoulders, your feet firmly planted about twelve inches apart

    b. Releasing tension by take several deep breaths and exhaling completely

    c. Feeling the earth beneath you supporting you and restoring your energy field

    d. Choosing to be fully present with your client, asking for spiritual guidance if necessary

10. Positive physiological responses to laughter include all of the following except (page 773)

    a. Releasing endorphins, giving us a sense of control and mastery of our circumstances

    b. Improving the immune system, eliminating cancerous cells, and promoting the release of neurotransmitters

    c. Helping mask uncomfortable or painful feelings

    d. Dampening corticosteroid production, avoiding immunosuppression

Friday Night at the Movies

33

The purpose of this chapter is to explore the concepts of psychiatric/mental health nursing through over one hundred films that present specific conditions, disorders, symptoms, and responses to mental health and illness. This review shows that mental stressors are not the exclusive property of the mentally ill—we all experience mental stressors, and the level of our mental health, as these movies show, determines our ability to cope with them. Moreover, taken together, the films form a general review of this textbook.

Reading Assignment

Please read Chapter 33, "Friday Night at the Movies," pages 779–799.

Key Terms

Don't forget to use the textbook's comprehensive Glossary, found on pages 831–840. Frequently using this tool will help you gain a professional working knowledge of the language of psychiatry and psychiatric nursing.

Exercises and Activities

1. Why do you think the authors chose Friday night for you to spend at the movies?

   _____

   _____

   _____

   _____

   _____

2. Go to the movies with a friend or colleague to see a film that has a theme related to psychiatric/mental health. Discuss the movie with your friend, based on your new knowledge of the concepts of this course. How did your reaction differ from that of your friend or colleague?

   _____

   _____

3. Rent a movie that will offer insight into an area of the course you find particularly puzzling or difficult. Which movie did you choose and why?

   _____

   _____

4. Go to the Online Companion for this book at www.DelmarNursing.com, and read about new movies with themes related to the content of this course. Which movies that you've never seen might be of particular interest to you?

    _____

    _____

5. Go to the Online Companion for this book at www.DelmarNursing.com, and tell other nursing students across the country about a movie you saw whose themes are applicable to the concepts taught in this course.

Comprehensive Practice
Final Examination

1. Neurotransmitters are (page 62)

   a. electrical signals in the brain.

   b. chemical messengers in the brain.

   c. neurons.

   d. synapses.

2. The current version of the American Psychiatric Association's Diagnostic and Statistical Manual is the (page 82)

   a. DSM-IIIR.

   b. DSM-IV.

   c. DSM-IV-TR

   d. DSM-V.

3. Axis IV of the DSM reflects (page 83)

   a. general psychiatric disorders.

   b. general medical disorders.

   c. psychosocial and environmental problems.

   d. global problems.

4. A surprising fact about NANDA's nursing diagnoses is (page 86)

   a. even though they are designed for use with clients who have any kind of health problem, over half of them pertain to psychosocial issues.

   b. someday the NANDA diagnoses will replace the DSM-IV.

   c. the NANDA diagnoses exclude human responses to mental disorders.

   d. the NANDA diagnoses will expire in the year 2000.

5. Defense mechanisms (page 103)

   a. refer to the immune system's ability to ward off disease.

   b. are inborn.

   c. protect people from mental illnesses.

   d. unconsciously protect people from internal conflicts and external stressors.

6. The Carter Commission (page 133)

    a. identified the "tip-of-the-iceberg" phenomenon.

    b. promoted deinstitutionalization.

    c. identified the prevalence and incidence of mental illnesses.

    d. made psychiatric nursing part of the general nursing curriculum.

7. Under all but the most dire circumstances, clients have the right to (pages 145–150)

    a. disrupt the treatment programs of other clients.

    b. smoke.

    c. refuse treatment.

    d. be judged by a panel of their peers.

8. To control violent or self-destructive behavior in clients, nurses are obligated to use (page 151)

    a. the least restrictive alternative.

    b. any means necessary.

    c. their best judgment.

    d. the physician's written order.

9. Hans Selye's General Adaptation Syndrome is (page 162)

    a. a medical diagnosis.

    b. a psychiatric diagnosis.

    c. a model of a healthy response to stress.

    d. irrelevant in some cultures.

10. The key difference between anxiety and fear is that (page 184)

    a. fear is normal, anxiety is not.

    b. fear is more often experienced by males, whereas anxiety is more often experienced by females.

    c. fear involves dread of some specific threat, whereas anxiety occurs without relation to a specific threat.

    d. fear is a nursing diagnosis, whereas anxiety is a medical diagnosis.

11. An appropriate intervention for someone seeking emergency care for acute stress would be (page 201)

    a. Assure the client that the future will be better

    b. Help the client cognitively reframe the stressful situation

    c. Sedation

    d. Meditation

12. Panic Disorder is (page 189)

    a. anxiety accompanied by crying.

    b. unrelated to anxiety.

    c. a form of anxiety characterized by intense episodes and specific physiological symptoms.

    d. anxiety accompanied by psychosis.

13. It is appropriate to diagnose Obsessive-Compulsive Disorder when (page 205)

    a. fear of self-contamination is consistent with risk.

    b. clients can't remember whether they turned off the oven.

    c. clients go through rituals.

    d. fear of self-contamination is inconsistent with risk.

14. Choice of treatment for anxiety depends on (page 200)

    a. The client's tolerance of drugs

    b. Whether the client uses alcohol or not

    c. The client's specific diagnosis

    d. The severity of the anxiety

15. Speech characterized by apparently random words that have no logical connection to one another is termed (page 219)

    a. neologizing.

    b. word salad.

    c. tangentiality.

    d. derailment.

16. The "positive" symptoms of schizophrenia include (page 223)

    a. hallucinations.

    b. flat affect.

    c. lack of relationships.

    d. withdrawal.

17. The "negative" symptoms of schizophrenia include (pages 224–225)

    a. disordered thought.

    b. delusions.

    c. anhedonia.

    d. bizarre behavior.

18. The dopamine hypothesis for schizophrenia suggests that (page 230)

    a. schizophrenia strikes at random.

    b. dopamine production is higher in the brains of people with schizophrenia.

    c. dopamine production is lower in the brains of people with schizophrenia.

    d. dopamine apparently has nothing to do with schizophrenia.

19. All of the following are true of neuroleptic medications except (page 233)

    a. Generally, most are more effective against the positive rather than the negative symptoms of schizophrenia

    b. Their mechanism often causes severe neuromuscular side effects

    c. They are the only treatment for schizophrenia that has proven effective

    d. They work by blocking dopamine, a neurotransmitter, at the brain's dopamine receptors

20. When a nurse has diagnosed a client with altered thought processes, the nurse should respond to the client by (page 236)

    a. redirecting the client's attention back to the here and now.

    b. exploring the client's delusions with him or her.

    c. arguing with the client about his or her disordered thoughts.

    d. speaking louder to be heard above the voices the client is hearing.

21. When planning care for clients in the rehabilitative phase of schizophrenia, the nurse should (page 237)

    a. allow the clients to spend time alone in a private space.

    b. give the clients responsibility for getting to their appointments on time.

    c. help the clients structure their day with a written schedule.

    d. befriend the client.

22. The difference between unipolar and bipolar depression is in (page 249)

    a. unipolar depression, the client is always hypomanic.

    b. unipolar depression, the client swings from one end of the mood continuum to the other.

    c. bipolar depression, the client has upswings, or highs, at least some of the time.

    d. bipolar depression, the client swings between depression and anxiety.

23. Symptoms of Major Depressive Disorder can include (page 250)

    a. hunger.

    b. thought disorder.

    c. suicidal thoughts.

    d. grandiosity.

24. The key difference between Major Depressive Disorder and Dysthymic Disorder is that (page 253)

    a. Dysthymic Disorder is just a short episode of depression.

    b. Dysthymic Disorder is a chronic depression lasting more than two years.

    c. Dysthymic Disorder is a depression brought on by a food allergy.

    d. Dysthymic Disorder is a side effect of psychotropic medications.

25. All of the following are normal stages of grief except (page 254)

    a. Recovery

    b. Reality

    c. Chronic

    d. Shock

26. Freud conceived the superego to be (page 257)

    a. the conscience.

    b. conceit.

    c. the supreme being.

    d. the cerebral cortex.

27. Classes of medications to treat depression include all of the following except (pages 260–263)

    a. MAO inhibitors.

    b. phenothiazines.

    c. tricyclics.

    d. selective serotonin reuptake inhibitors.

28. For planning the nursing care of clients with depression, nurses may find it useful to think in terms of Orem's Self-Care Deficit Theory because (page 264)

    a. depressed clients usually can't take care of themselves.

    b. nurses need to take over the care of clients with depression

    c. clients with depressions need to be expected to take care of themselves.

    d. the self-care of clients with depression needs to be thoughtfully planned.

29. The key difference between mania and hypomania is that (page 282)

    a. the number and length of manic behaviors are fewer and shorter in hypomania.

    b. there is no difference.

    c. unlike mania, hypomania is not a DSM-IV diagnosis and is very similar to general happiness.

    d. mania includes psychosis, whereas hypomania does not.

30. The transition from mania to depression or depression to mania is called (page 282)

    a. cyclothymic patterns.

    b. Bipolar Disorder.

    c. the switch process.

    d. manic-depressive illness.

31. Strong evidence suggests Bipolar Disorder is caused by (page 284)

    a. genetic factors.

    b. environmental factors.

    c. developmental factors.

    d. learned behavior.

32. All of the following can produce symptoms similar to mania except (pages 286–288)

    a. Drugs

    b. Physical diseases

    c. Sleep deprivation

    d. Financial difficulties

33. Drugs that can cause switching from a depressive episode to a manic state include all of the following except (page 286)

    a. lithium.

    b. anabolic steroids.

    c. tricyclic antidepressants.

    d. St. John's Wort.

34. All of the following reasons contribute to noncompliance on the part of clients prescribed lithium except (pages 290–291)

    a. Lithium is ineffective in eliminating mood swings

    b. Lithium can cloud cognitive functioning

    c. Lithium is embryotoxic in the first trimester

    d. Physical side effects can include hypothyroidsim, kidney problems, and nervous system symptoms

35. The primary treatment for Bipolar Disorder is (page 292)

    a. psychotherapy.

    b. electroconvulsive therapy (ECT).

    c. medications.

    d. behavioral therapy.

36. A nursing intervention effective with clients who are manic is to (page 296)

    a. challenge the client's intrusive behavior and racing thoughts.

    b. use group therapy.

    c. urge the client to get more sleep.

    d. reduce unnecessary stimulation in the therapeutic environment.

37. An example of tertiary prevention of suicide might be (page 320)

    a. removing sharp or dangerous objects from the environment.

    b. assessing clients for suicide risk.

    c. learning CPR and other emergency medical procedures.

    d. monitoring clients closely.

38. An effective intervention nurses can use to lower the risk of clients committing suicide would be (page 322)

    a. keeping a watchful eye.

    b. establishing a suicide contract with clients to ensure safety for a specific period of time.

    c. hoping your relationship is strong enough with clients that they wouldn't commit suicide while you are on duty.

    d. healing touch.

39. A strong indicator of dependence on a substance or drug would be that the client (page 332)

    a. has used an addictive substance.

    b. uses the substance secretively.

    c. frequents places where substances are frequently abused.

    d. tries unsuccessfully to stop using a substance.

40. The CAGE questionnaire is used to (page 339)

    a. assess for claustrophobia.

    b. count words-per-minute for a person experiencing mania.

    c. detect alcoholism.

    d. determine type of substance abused.

41. Opiates are powerfully addicting substances because they (page 348)

    a. fit perfectly into endorphin receptors.

    b. can be taken by many different routes of administration.

    c. are highly concentrated psychoactive substances.

    d. have been accepted in general use for many generations.

42. Methadone maintenance as a treatment for heroine addiction works because (page 348)

    a. it prevents withdrawal symptoms while blocking the pleasurable effects of opiates, allowing the client to function without drug euphoria.

    b. many addicts divert methadone to the street while secretly taking opiates.

    c. it enables addicts to substitute one street drug for another.

    d. it enables addicts to practice behaviors associated with drug use.

43. The principal danger of using hallucinogens is (page 349)

    a. dangerous behavior due to poor judgment or faulty perceptions.

    b. addiction or dependence.

    c. they lead to the use of other drugs.

    d. never returning to normal.

44. Up to 50% of people who abuse drugs (page 350)

    a. abuse more than one drug and/or have another psychiatric diagnosis.

    b. are women.

    c. are in prison.

    d. have a major medical disorder.

45. Codependence refers to (page 352)

    a. the phenomenon of being dependent on two or more drugs at one time.

    b. two people sharing a substance dependence.

    c. the relationship between a substance abuser and a significant other who facilitates the substance abuse.

    d. the relationship between a substance abuser and a spouse abuser.

46. A personality disorder manifests itself in (page 365)

    a. old age.

    b. infancy.

    c. adolescence and early adulthood.

    d. early childhood.

47. Personality disorders are classified as Axis II disorders in the DSM-IV because (page 365)

    a. major psychiatric disorders on Axis I are constant across all personality types.

    b. people with personality disorders don't have major psychiatric disorders like those on Axis I.

    c. Axis II disorders color Axis I disorders.

    d. a and c

48. Antisocial Personality Disorder is classified as one the following groups of personality disorders: (page 374)

    a. Anxiety and fear-based group

    b. Odd and eccentric group

    c. Dramatic and emotional group

    d. None of these

49. In Borderline Personality Disorder, the term *borderline* was coined because the client is living on the border between (page 368)

    a. schizophrenia and depression.

    b. anxiety and mania.

    c. psychosis and neurosis.

    d. sanity and insanity.

50. People with Narcissistic Personality Disorder are probably overrepresented in the psychiatric care community because they (page 371)

    a. want to be the center of attention.

    b. have difficulty forming relationships.

    c. have difficulty dealing with life stressors.

    d. are predominantly female and have fewer problems seeking help.

51. To individuals with Antisocial Personality Disorder, a nurse is (page 376)

    a. a person who can help them transcend the disorder.

    b. an obstacle to being able to pursue their ends.

    c. a means to an end, like everybody else.

    d. someone with whom they can form a meaningful relationship.

52. Although people with Schizotypal Personality Disorder share many cognitive attributes with people who have schizophrenia, people with Schizoid Personality Disorder (page 379)

    a. have almost all the cognitive attributes of schizophrenia.

    b. resemble anxious people.

    c. appear as just plain odd.

    d. have long periods of normal behavior interrupted by periods of Schizoid Personality Disorder.

53. People experiencing a Paranoid Personality Disorder are different from people experiencing schizophrenia of the paranoid type in that people with (page 381)

    a. Paranoid Personality Disorder can lash out violently toward a person who makes them feel threatened, whereas people with schizophrenia are unlikely to be violent when provoked by acute feelings of paranoia toward a person.

    b. Paranoid Personality Disorder are more likely to experience hallucinations whereas people with schizophrenia of the paranoid type are more likely to have delusions.

    c. schizophrenia of the paranoid type are psychotic, whereas people with Paranoid Personality Disorder are not likely to be psychotic.

    d. schizophrenia of the paranoid type are likely to be paranoid all the time, whereas people with Paranoid Personality Disorder are likely to be paranoid only occasionally.

54. The best nursing approach toward clients with odd or eccentric personality disorders is to (page 383)

    a. draw the clients' attention to the cognitive aspects of their disorders.

    b. focus on relationship-building.

    c. minimize or dismiss disturbing or bizarre thoughts.

    d. give the clients feedback on their behavior.

55. Compared to Obsessive-Compulsive Disorder (OCD), Obsessive-Compulsive Personality Disorder (OCPD) (page 384)

    a. involves behavior in response to highly specific stimuli.

    b. is a pervasive disorder that encompasses every aspect of its victim's life.

    c. tends to disappear toward midlife.

    d. sufferers have more insight into their disorder than people suffering from OCD.

56. The person with Avoidant Personality Disorder tries to avoid (page 386)

    a. anything that would tend to raise the person's visibility.

    b. responsibility.

    c. immediate family members and close friends.

    d. familiar surroundings.

57. A person with a Dependent Personality Disorder has a need to be cared for by others. Also characteristic of a person with this disorder is (page 388)

    a. indecisiveness.

    b. strong opinions.

    c. unusual maturity.

    d. highly risky behavior.

58. Another name for Passive-Aggressive Personality Disorder is (page 388)

    a. Maddening Personality Disorder.

    b. Negativistic Personality Disorder.

    c. Antisocial Personality Disorder.

    d. Mother-in-law syndrome.

59. Regardless of the type of personality disorder, which of the following statements is true? (page 390)

    a. We all have these disorders sooner or later.

    b. These are extremely common disorders affecting a large percentage of the population.

    c. Personality disorders are highly treatable.

    d. Personality disorders are characterized by pervasive personality traits that seriously impair their victims' ability to function.

60. Research shows that nurses respond least empathically to clients who are diagnosed with (page 369)

    a. Borderline Personality Disorder.

    b. Antisocial Personality Disorder.

    c. schizophrenia.

    d. Bipolar Disorder.

61. Clients with Somatization Disorder (page 403)

    a. have a physical disease and don't know it.

    b. don't have a physical disease and don't know it.

    c. have a physical disease and know it.

    d. don't have a physical disease but are convinced they do.

62. Although cognitive-behavioral therapy may be helpful to people with Somatization Disorder, an obstacle to its effectiveness is (page 406)

    a. it usually only works in combination with medication therapy.

    b. "Cures" of physical disabilities are greeted with skepticism.

    c. it can take years for improvements

    d. clients won't accept it because they don't believe there is a psychological component to their illness.

63. The best approach for nurses to take toward people with Hypochondriasis is to (page 409)

    a. as with other psychiatric disorders in which clients imagine fears not based on reality, ignore the clients' concerns about their physical health and concentrate on psychosocial issues.

    b. recommend an intensive physical work-up.

    c. emphasize the clients' general good health and put symptoms in the context of being real and troublesome, not imaginary or dangerous.

    d. identify any other psychiatric disorder the clients may have and focus on the alternate diagnosis.

64. The key difference between conversion reaction and a Factitious Disorder is that (page 409)

    a. the cause of conversion reaction is psychological, whereas the source of Factitious Disorder is antisocial.

    b. the cause of conversion reaction is physical, whereas the source of Factitious Disorder is psychological.

    c. conversion reaction is a somatoform disorder, whereas Factitious Disorder arises from personality disorders.

    d. people with conversion reaction believe they are physically ill, whereas people with Factitious Disorder know deep down inside that they are not.

65. The appropriate response of a nurse to people with Factitious Disorder is to (page 412)

    a. help the clients recognize that, with current limitations on the resources of the health care system, health professionals cannot be squandering these resources on people who feign illness.

    b. recognize that, in their own unique way, people with Factitious Disorder are as much in need of psychiatric care as people with other psychiatric disorders.

    c. redirect those who feign illness to practitioners who feign cures.

    d. recommend vigorous interventions to satisfy clients who present themselves as ill.

66. Primary insomnia is only considered a psychiatric disorder if (page 424)

    a. it lasts a month and interferes with a person's functioning.

    b. it is a consequence of some other psychiatric disorder.

    c. it has an organic cause.

    d. the client defines it as a psychiatric disorder.

67. Nurses can teach clients to improve sleep hygiene by recommending that they (page 426)

    a. restrict the bedroom to sleep and sexual activity only.

    b. eat a heavy meal before retiring.

    c. have an alcoholic beverage before retiring.

    d. rise when the sun rises and retire when the sun sets.

68. Narcolepsy is (page 428)

   a. the opposite of sleepwalking.

   b. a side effect of addiction to narcotics.

   c. a rare disorder that may run in families, characterized by sleep attacks accompanied by cataplexy or hallucinations.

   d. a fictitious disorder made up by writers.

69. The key difference's between nightmares and sleep terrors include all the following except (page 428)

   a. Nightmare Disorder is a DSM-IV diagnosis, whereas there is no such DSM-IV Disorder as sleep terror disorder.

   b. clients can remember the content of nightmares but they cannot remember the content of sleep terrors.

   c. nightmares often require an extensive diagnostic work-up in a sleep disorders clinic, whereas the diagnosis of sleep terrors is relatively straightforward.

   d. they are the same things.

70. Developing a positive body image is important to adolescents. Nurses can promote a positive body image by teaching adolescents the "Three As," which include all the following except (page 433)

   a. Accept yourself for what you are

   b. Attention: Feed, rest, and exercise your body based on the cues it gives you

   c. Apprehension or Alarm: Be able to recognize when your body is getting too fat

   d. Appreciation: Enjoy your body for the pleasure and safety if provides

71. The key difference between Bulimia Nervosa and Anorexia Nervosa is that (page 433)

   a. people with anorexia have a distorted body image that impels them to continue losing weight to a point where their body develops dangerous medical conditions; people with bulimia just use bingeing and purging as dysfunctional means of weight control.

   b. bulimia is generally treated outside the hospital; once the client is admitted to the hospital for treatment, the diagnosis becomes anorexia.

   c. people with bulimia use fasting, bingeing, and purging as means of weight control; people with anorexia use fasting and exercising.

   d. bulimia is episodic, whereas anorexia is a long-term diagnosis.

72. Hypoactive Sexual Desire Disorder is most frequently caused by (page 441)

    a. advancing age.

    b. hormonal abnormalities.

    c. relationship problems.

    d. gender identity problems.

73. All of the following are DSM-IV diagnoses related to sexuality and gender identity except (page 445)

    a. Homosexuality

    b. Gender identity

    c. Premature ejaculation

    d. Exhibitionism

74. Knowledge and skills necessary for nurses to effectively manage pain in their clients include all of the following except

    a. political and administrative skills to ensure that clients receive the best possible care.

    b. advanced practice certification.

    c. knowledge of pharmacology.

    d. knowledge of the neurobiology of pain

75. The main role of the liaison psychiatric nurse is to (page 471)

    a. keep the psychiatrist informed of his or her clients' developments while they are hospitalized for physical conditions.

    b. provide consultation and teaching to medical nurses when a client with a psychiatric condition is being treated in a medical unit.

    c. handle the questions from clients' families.

    d. provide psychiatric care to clients who are physically ill.

76. Psychoneuroimmunology is a field that seeks to (page 473)

    a. find the physical causes of stress.

    b. understand the biological basis for mental illnesses.

    c. understand the mind-body connection.

    d. find ways to boost the body's ability to withstand stress.

77. All of the following contributed to massive deinstitutionalization of people with chronic or severe mental illnesses in the late 1960s and 1970s except (page 480)

   a. Concern for the civil rights of people with mental illnesses

   b. Desire for cost cutting

   c. Full commitment to mental health treatment and support services in the community

   d. Significant improvements in the medications available to treat mental disorders

78. Just as there are "childhood" diseases among the physical diseases, there are also "childhood" disorders among the mental illnesses. Mental disorders unique to childhood include all of the following except (page 495)

   a. Personality disorders

   b. Autistic Disorder

   c. Conduct Disorder

   d. Attention-Deficit Hyperactivity Disorder

79. Nurses should be alert to the following dynamics of childhood depression except (page 500)

   a. Many traditional clinicians don't believe children experience depression

   b. Childhood depression may manifest itself as irritable or aggressive behavior

   c. Depressed children become delusional

   d. Depression in children may be related to neglect or abuse

80. All of the following nursing skills are useful in assessing the mental health of a child except (page 508)

   a. Family assessment skills

   b. Play therapy

   c. Developmental assessment knowledge

   d. Psychodrama

81. Asperger's Syndrome differs from Autism in that (page 506)

    a. Asperger's does not lead to social isolation.

    b. Asperger's is treatable.

    c. Asperger's is characterized by repetitive actions or behaviors.

    d. Asperger's is associated with no known neurological abnormalities.

82. The healthiest form of identify formation in adolescents is (page 523)

    a. identity achievement.

    b. Foreclosure.

    c. moratorium.

    d. identity diffusion.

83. Adolescence is an age group at high risk for suicide. Signs that should raise concerns about an increased risk for suicide include all of the following except (page 533)

    a. Increase in impulsive behavior

    b. Giving away cherished belongings

    c. Decreased appetite

    d. Preoccupation with death and dying

84. The factor that most protects teenagers from engaging in dangerous risk-taking behaviors is (page 535)

    a. authoritarian parenting style.

    b. connectedness with parents and school.

    c. strong spiritual beliefs.

    d. peer group.

85. Actions nurses can take to help develop a therapeutic relationship with an adolescent include all of the following except (page 536)

    a. Adopt interests and lifestyle choices currently popular with adolescents

    b. Self-disclose information as a means validating an adolescent's experience

    c. Help adolescents identify their strengths and reasons for positive self-image

    d. Listen actively

86. Signs and symptoms of dementia include all of the following except (page 553)

    a. Paranoia.

    b. Disinhibition.

    c. Wandering.

    d. Reminiscing.

87. Ways nurses can assist fatigued caretakers of elderly friends and relatives with dementia include (page 579)

    a. suggesting clients' physicians order or increase sedatives.

    b. assisting caregivers in planning alternate care arrangements in a guilt-free manner consistent with the clients' best interests.

    c. encouraging caregivers to discuss their fatigue frankly with clients.

    d. helping caregivers accept their fatigue and stress.

88. Nurses are obligated to take all of the following actions in response to a client who is the victim of child abuse or rape except (page 590)

    a. Nurses must report child abuse or rape to the appropriate authorities.

    b. Nurses should know how to maintain the integrity of any evidence needed to prosecute a crime.

    c. Nurses should understand the dynamics of abuse and examine their own feelings toward these issues.

    d. Nurses should treat these cases like any other physical injury that has psychosocial implications.

89. Atypical neuroleptics are gaining wide acceptance in the treatment of psychosis because they are (page 639)

    a. cheaper than haloperidol and other phenathiazines.

    b. preferred by clients who want the latest treatments.

    c. safe for children under 18.

    d. relatively free of extra-pyramidal side effects.

90. Prescribing stimulants is controversial because these drugs are easily abused and their effectiveness is either unproven or heatedly debated, except for the treatment of (page 663)

    a. Attention-Deficit Disorder.

    b. anxiety.

    c. Obsessive-Compulsive Personality Disorder.

    d. narcolepsy.

91. All of the following statements about psychoanalysis are true except (page 672)

    a. Its techniques and insights remain useful today

    b. It is an expensive, lengthy form of therapy that insurance does not usually cover and few individuals can afford

    c. It is only effective in treating schizophrenia

    d. It has given way to shorter, more cost-effective forms of individual therapy

92. Cognitive-behavioral therapy (page 674)

    a. offers insight into the childhood origins of adult problems.

    b. works by allowing clients to "talk through" their problems.

    c. offers solutions to problems that actively involve making behavioral changes.

    d. is similar to psychoanalysis in the cost and length of treatment.

93. Nurses find it useful to view families as systems because (page 687)

    a. families are less than the sum of their parts (individuals).

    b. dysfunctions cannot produce equilibria.

    c. the changes affecting an individual have an effect on the whole family.

    d. other parts of society work like systems.

94. The trifocal model refers to (page 729)

    a. individual, family, and community.

    b. wellness, prevention, and problem intervention.

    c. medicine, nursing, and allied health.

    d. id, ego, and superego.

95. When a nursing diagnosis of caregiver role strain has been established, it is important for the nurse to (page 745)

   a. give the stressed caregiver regular breaks.

   b. teach the caregiver more about caring models.

   c. recognize the ways in which the caregiver adds to his or her own strain.

   d. include the caregiver in the health care planning team.

96. Ecomaps are a useful way to (page 685)

   a. assess the genetic component of diseases in the family.

   b. identify the person in the family with the greatest psychic strength.

   c. understand family dynamics.

   d. develop nursing care plans.

97. Group therapy is a good way to (page 713)

   a. get withdrawn clients to talk.

   b. make clients feel that they are not alone, that others share their problems.

   c. get better compliance on the unit, due to the collaborative decision making.

   d. elicit extremely personal revelations.

98. Capitation is a funding mechanism that (page 728)

   a. cuts off claimants.

   b. establishes a single payment for a particular kind of disorder, like mental disorders, for a specific period of time to limit the insurer's liability.

   c. identifies coverages or clients the insurance company won't cover.

   d. charges a "per head" fee for services as they are delivered.

99. Relaxation techniques and guided imagery are examples of treatment modalities that are (pages 745–748)

   a. complementary, or adjunct, to other psychiatric treatment modalities.

   b. inappropriate to nursing practice.

   c. not proven to be ineffective.

   d. harmful, not helpful.

100. Centering is a nursing self-care modality that (page 762)

    a. once learned, takes only 30 to 60 seconds to perform.

    b. helps the nurse focus on the work immediately ahead.

    c. releases tension, placing the nurse fully in the present.

    d. All of the above

Answers to Self-Assessment Quizzes

Chapter 1:
Through the Door: Your First Day in Psychiatric Nursing

1. T
2. T
3. b
4. c
5. d
6. d
7. c
8. d
9. "Rites of passage" might be defined as an experience that marks a significant event, achievement, pathway, or growth.
10. "Being present" could be defined as caring, listening, affirming, and responding to or supporting clients, often in nurturing, nonverbal ways.

Chapter 2:
Psychiatric Nursing: The Evolution of a Specialty

1. F
2. T
3. F
4. T
5. F
6. a
7. b
8. b, a, d, g, e, c, f
9. f, g, a, d, b, c, e

Chapter 3:
Theory as A Basis for Practic

1. T
2. F
3. T
4. T
5. T
6. T
7. T
8. Relationships
9. Modeling
10. Leininger, Watson, and/or Boyken & Schoenhofer
11. Energy Fields
12. Self-Care Deficit
13. Id, Ego, and Superego
14. Erikson
15. Social or interpersonal
16. Cognitive
17. Behavioral
18. a

Chapter 4:
Neuroscience as Basis for Practice

1. T
2. F
3. T
4. T
5. T

6. T
7. T
8. Relationships
9. Modeling
10. Leininger, Watson, and/or Boykin and Schoenhofer
11. Energy fields
12. Self-care deficit
13. Id, ego, and superego
14. Erikson
15. Social or interpersonal
16. Cognitive
17. Behavioral
18. d
19. d
20. c
21. c

Chapter 5:
Diagnostic Systems
for Psychiatric Nursing

1. F
2. T
3. F
4. T
5. F
6. F
7. T
8. T
9. F
10. F
11. T

Chapter 6:
Tools of Psychiatric
Mental Health Nursing

1. d
2. d
3. c
4. d
5. d
6. d
7. c
8. b
9. c
10. b

Chapter 7:
Cultural and Ethnic Considerations

1. F
2. F
3. T
4. T
5. T
6. a
7. e
8. d
9. b
10. a

Chapter 8:
Epidemiology of
Mental Health and Illness

1. T
2. T
3. T

4. T

5. F

6. f

7. c

8. a

9. b

10. d

Chapter 9:
Ethical and Legal Bases for Care

1. F

2. T

3. F

4. T

5. T

6. a

7. c

8. a

9. c

10. b

Chapter 10:
The Client Undergoing Crisis

1. T

2. F

3. T

4. T

5. T

6. c

7. c

8. d

9. c

10. b

Chapter 11:
The Client Experiencing Anxiety

1. T

2. T

3. F

4. F

5. F

6. c

7. d

8. c

9. a

10. c

Chapter 12:
The Client Experiencing Schizophrenia

1. F

2. T

3. T

4. T

5. F

6. T

7. F

8. F

9. F

10. T

11. T

12. F

13. F

14. F

15. F

16. T

17. d

18. c and f

19. c

20. b

Chapter 13:
The Client Experiencing Depression

1. F

2. T

3. T

4. T

5. T

6. T

7. T

8. F

9. a

10. b

11. a

12. b

13. c

14. d

15. a

Chapter 14:
The Client Experiencing Mania

1. T

2. F

3. T

4. T

5. F

6. F

7. b

8. a

9. d

10. c

11. c

12. c

Chapter 15:
The Client Who Is Suicidal

1. F

2. T

3. T

4. F

5. F

6. a

7. a

8. a

9. a

10. d

Chapter 16:
The Client Who Abuses
Chemical Substances

1. T

2. T

3. T

4. F

5. F

6. c

7. c

8. c

9. a

10. d

Chapter 17:
The Client with a Personality Disorder

1. F

2. T

3. T

4. T

5. T

6. d

7. c

8. a

9. c

10. d

Chapter 18:
The Client Experiencing
a Somatoform Disorder

1. F

2. T

3. T

4. T

5. T

6. d

7. c

8. c

9. e

10. c

Chapter 19:
The Client with Disorders
of Self-Regulation

1. F

2. F

3. T

4. T

5. T

6. a

7. g

8. a

9. c

10. a

Chapter 20:
The Physically Ill Client
Experiencing Emotional Distress

1. T

2. F

3. T

4. T

5. F

6. c

7. a

8. c

9. c

10. b

Chapter 21:
Forgotten Populations

1. T

2. T

3. F

4. T

5. F

6. T

7. T

8. a

9. c

10. a

Chapter 22:
The Child

1. T

2. F

3. T

4. T

5. T

6. b

7. a

8. c

9. a

10. a

Chapter 23:
The Adolescent

1. T

2. T

3. F

4. T

5. F

6. T

7. c

8. b

9. c

10. a

11. a

Chapter 24:
The Elderly

1. T

2. T

3. F

4. T

5. F

6. a

7. b

8. c

9. c

10. a

Chapter 25:
Survivors of Violence or Abuse

1. T

2. F

3. F

4. F

5. T

6. b

7. a

8. c

9. b

10. d

Chapter 26:
Pharmacology in Psychiatric Care

1. T

2. T

3. F

4. T

5. F

6. T

7. d

8. c

9. d

10. b

11. c

12. P

D

P

A

A

A

P

D

D

P

A

P

A

P

Chapter 27:
Individual Psychotherapy

1. T
2. F
3. F
4. T
5. T
6. b
7. a
8. c
9. a
10. c

Chapter 28:
Family Therapy

1. F
2. T
3. T
4. F
5. F
6. d
7. c
8. a
9. c
10. b

Chapter 29:
Group Therapy

1. T
2. T
3. T
4. F
5. T
6. d
7. c
8. a
9. c
10. c

Chapter 30:
Community Mental Health Nursing

1. T
2. T
3. T
4. F
5. F
6. c
7. d
8. b
9. b
10. b

Chapter 31:
Complementary and Somatic Therapies

1. T
2. T
3. F
4. T
5. F

6. a

7. b

8. c

9. c

10. a

Chapter 32: Self-Care Modalities

1. F

2. T

3. T

4. T

5. F

6. c

7. d

8. d

9. a

10. c

Answers to Comprehensive Practice Final Examination

1. b		30. c	
2. b		31. a	
3. c		32. d	
4. a		33. b	
5. d		34. a	
6. c		35. c	
7. c		36. d	
8. a		37. c	
9. c		38. b	
10. c		39. d	
11. b		40. c	
12. c		41. a	
13. d		42. a	
14. b		43. d	
15. b		44. a	
16. a		45. c	
17. c		46. c	
18. b		47. d	
19. c		48. c	
20. a		49. c	
21. c		50. c	
22. c		51. c	
23. c		52. c	
24. b		53. c	
25. d		54. d	
26. a		55. b	
27. b		56. a	
28. d		57. a	
29. a		58. b	

59. d		80. d	
60. a		81. d	
61. d		82. b	
62. d		83. c	
63. c		84. a	
64. d		85. b	
65. b		86. d	
66. a		87. b	
67. a		88. d	
68. c		89. a	
69. b		90. d	
70. c		91. c	
71. a		92. c	
72. c		93. c	
73. a		94. b	
74. a		95. d	
75. b		96. c	
76. c		97. b	
77. c		98. b	
78. a		99. a	
79. a		100. d	